The F.
Rep

. . . .

. . . . . .

DO NOT REMOVE
CARDS FROM POCKET

OTHER BOOKS FROM
THE PEOPLE'S MEDICAL SOCIETY

Getting the Most for Your Medical Dollar

Massage Made Easy

Medicare Made Easy

Medicine on Trial

Misdiagnosis: Woman As a Disease

So You're Going to Be a Mother

Take This Book to the Gynecologist With You

Take This Book to the Hospital With You

Take This Book to the Pediatrician With You

The Complete Book of Relaxation Techniques

Yoga Made Easy

Your Medical Rights

The Hormone Replacement Handbook

Paula Brisco and Karla Morales

≡People's Medical Society®

Allentown, Pennsylvania

The People's Medical Society is a nonprofit consumer health organization dedicated to the principles of better, more responsive and less expensive medical care. Organized in 1983, the People's Medical Society puts previously unavailable medical information into the hands of consumers so that they can make informed decisions about their own health care.

Membership in the People's Medical Society is $20 a year and includes a subscription to the *People's Medical Society Newsletter.* For information, write to the People's Medical Society, 462 Walnut Street, Allentown, PA 18102, or call 610-770-1670.

This and other People's Medical Society publications are available for quantity purchase at discount. Contact the People's Medical Society for details.

Many of the designations used by manufacturers and sellers to distinguish their products are claimed as trademarks. Where those designations appear in this book and the People's Medical Society was aware of a trademark claim, the designations have been printed in initial capital letters (e.g., Premarin).

© 1996 by the People's Medical Society
Printed in the United States of America

Library of Congress Cataloging-in-Publication Data
Brisco, Paula.
    The hormone replacement handbook / by Paula Brisco and
Karla Morales.
      p. cm.
    Includes bibliographical references and index.
    ISBN 1-882606-20-5
    1. Menopause—Hormone therapy. I. Morales, Karla. II. Title.
RG186.B75 1996
618.1'75061—dc20   95-50266
                                                         CIP

1 2 3 4 5 6 7 8 9 0
First printing, January 1996

CONTENTS

CHAPTER III

HRT and the Treatment of Menopausal Symptoms

CHAPTER IV

Preventive Hormone Therapy After Menopause

CHAPTER VII

Weighing Your Choices 195

Controversy surrounds women's health. Sometimes the controversy is due to medical excess. For example, most medical researchers say that the majority of cesarean-section surgery is unnecessary. The same is noted for hysterectomies. Other times the controversy is about what is lacking. The dearth of genuine medical research on women and heart disease is only one example of a long list of health research that has paid scant attention to women.

But probably the most controversial issue swirling around women's health in the 1990s is hormone replacement therapy (HRT). As Paula Brisco and Karla Morales point out in this most important book, HRT is a "treatment" for menopause that leaves a lot of questions unanswered. It is a relatively new therapy, but a very common one. By some it is heralded as a "cure" for menopause. By others it's called dangerous. Some tout the positive side effects of HRT such as increased protection against heart disease. Others worry about the possible increase in the risk of breast cancer.

While there are many books about menopause, we were struck by the lack of material available to the consumer about hormone replacement therapy. Even though HRT is the number one prescribed treatment for menopausal symptoms, most women know little more than what their physicians know or tell them. More often than not that information is just not enough. To make a fully informed decision, a woman needs all the available data presented in a way that is easy to understand and clearly presented.

The challenge of this book was to review all the research that has been done on hormone replacement therapy and present it in a way that you, the reader, can come to some conclusions. It would have been easy to write a book and give one side and downplay the other. In fact, most books on health do that. However, at the People's Medical Society, our goal has always been to gather the data, present the facts to you and let you make the decision. That was clearly the objective in this book.

Some readers will go away from this book ready to use HRT. Others will say never. Some women will be introduced to alternatives to HRT presented in this book. Others may have already tried those remedies and will want more. Certain readers will end up having more questions than when they started. That cannot be helped. It merely illustrates how personal and controversial the use of HRT is.

As new and more technically involved medical therapies come along, the list of questions and doubts grows. For the consumer this means the need to be more and better informed. Before you make any medical decision, it is essential that you know the facts, opinions, controversies and available alternatives. It is also important to recognize that the decision is yours. It is not a decision for your practitioner to make—although a good practitioner will be your partner in health. It is not what your friends tell you—what works for them may not work for you. It is truly up to you.

While Paula Brisco and Karla Morales cannot take the controversy out of hormone replacement therapy, they certainly have taken the mystery out of it. I am confident that you will find this to be the most helpful resource you use in making the decision about whether hormone replacement therapy is for you.

Charles B. Inlander
President
People's Medical Society

The Hormone
Replacement Handbook

Aside from bulleted lists, boldfaced terms are found in the glossary, beginning on page 221. Only the first mention of the word in the text will be boldfaced.

We have tried to use male and female pronouns in an egalitarian manner throughout the book. Any imbalance in usage has been in the interest of readability.

The Raging Hormone Debate

The fact that you have this book in your hands shows that you are one of the many women who are evaluating **hormone replacement therapy (HRT)**. Perhaps you have begun **menopause**, and your doctor has suggested HRT. Perhaps you have a family history of **osteoporosis**, and you've heard that HRT can prevent the disease. Maybe your thoughts of HRT began with a conversation with friends and family members. Or maybe you are looking ahead to health issues that may affect you in five or 10 years.

Regardless of the reason you find yourself here, you join the ranks of millions of women who, at some time in their lives, are faced with the decision whether to take hormone replacement therapy or not.

You may find that making the decision is clear-cut. Most women, however, find that the issue is complicated by the fact that there is, as of yet, no consensus in the medical field about the best uses of HRT. Clinical studies continue to evaluate its pros and cons. As new evidence comes to light, you and your health care practitioner can use these data to make an informed choice for or against hormone replacement.

HRT raises issues about American health care in general. Are we treating menopause as a disease instead of as a natural stage of the body's life span, and if so, is that approach correct? Is the medical profession rushing to promote a therapy that may have unknown side effects 20 or 30 years down the road? Is it wise to tout HRT for all women when only certain women may need it?

The HRT Basics

Before we can address these issues—which are the thrust of this book—we need to define our terms. We've mentioned the word **hormone:** What exactly does that mean? A hormone is a complex chemical secreted by certain glands in the body. The hormone travels through the bloodstream and controls the action of a specific organ or group of cells. The growth hormone, for example, controls the growth of bones in the body. In the female body, the hormone **estrogen** is one of several hormones that controls the reproductive process.

If hormones are natural chemicals, what, then, is hormone replacement therapy?

HRT is a medical treatment designed to supplement and/or replace the hormone estrogen that is produced in smaller and smaller amounts during and after menopause. HRT is also known by several other names: estrogen therapy (ET), **estrogen replacement therapy (ERT)** and combined hormone therapy (CHT).

Women often use the words "change of life" to describe

menopause; doctors may call it the climacteric. What exactly is it? Menopause is a medical term that signifies the normal and complete cessation of menstrual cycles, including both **ovulation** (the release of an egg from the **ovary**) and menstrual periods. In this usage, menopause is a discrete, one-time event: a woman's last menstrual period. In everyday usage, however, the word menopause can refer to the months before and the years after the last period. In this book you will find the word used in both senses, although more frequently in the latter sense.

Menopause is an inevitable phase of life. Every woman will eventually experience it unless her life is cut short. Menopause usually takes place between the ages of 45 and 55, although some women experience their last period in their 60s, and others in their 30s. You will probably have signals that you are approaching menopause. Disrupted menstrual cycles and irregular periods are common flags of its onset.

The menstrual cycle halts when the female body no longer produces enough estrogen. Estrogen is primarily a female or feminizing hormone—although men do produce it in much smaller amounts.

Speaking scientifically the word *estrogen* is a generic term. There are actually three types of estrogen. The first estrogen, **estradiol**, is manufactured by the ovaries and is the most potent form of estrogen. Estradiol is a part of the intricate biological system that results in the normal monthly ovulatory cycle. **Estrone**, a low-level estrogen, is made in the body's fatty tissues. Although produced at much lower levels than estradiol, estrone plays a role in building strong bones both before and after menopause. The third estrogen, **estriol**, is relatively weak and is generated when estradiol and estrone are used in the body.

What exactly is the role of estrogen in the female body? As a group, the three estrogens have fundamental tasks. First, estrogens function in the development of the breasts, ovaries and **uterus** from the time of adolescence through the reproductive years. Second, estrogens function in the menstrual cycle itself. (We will look at the latter function in greater detail in Chapter 2.)

Estrogen affects other areas of the body, too. The tissues in the **cervix**, **vagina** and bladder are sensitive to estrogen levels in the bloodstream. Estrogen helps your bones to absorb calcium, keeping bone mass high and bones strong. And in the blood itself, estrogen raises the levels of **HDL (high-density lipoprotein)** cholesterol, the so-called good cholesterol, while lowering the levels of **LDL (low-density lipoprotein)**, the "bad" cholesterol.

Estrogen is assisted by **progesterone**, another female sex hormone produced by the ovaries. In the process of reproduction, estrogen's primary task is to build up the lining of the uterus to receive a fertilized egg. If an egg is fertilized, progesterone prepares the uterus to accept the egg so that it can grow. If the egg is unfertilized, progesterone assists in shedding the uterine lining, which causes normal bleeding known as menstruation.

What Will HRT Achieve?

There are persuasive reasons to take hormone replacement therapy beginning at the time of menopause. They include:

To combat menopausal symptoms. Hot flashes, excessive sweating, vaginal dryness, irregular or prolonged periods and other classic symptoms of menopause can be allayed or deferred with HRT. We say deferred because in women who take HRT for short periods of time (a few years, for instance), these menopausal symptoms will recur when HRT is discontinued. (We will detail these symptoms in Chapter 3.)

To combat atrophy (shrinking of the tissues). Without estrogen, tissues in the vagina, bladder, muscles, breasts and skin begin to lose their resilience. In some women this situation gradually leads to more frequent vaginal and urinary infections, decreasing muscle strength, sagging breasts and drier and looser skin. By replenishing the body with estrogen through HRT, vaginal and urinary infections are less likely to occur, muscle tone is easier to maintain and, although estrogen doesn't prevent aging and wrinkling, it helps maintain a cushion of oil-producing collagen under the skin, making it seem more flexible and younger.

To combat loss of bone mass. Estrogen helps the bone absorb calcium. When estrogen is absent from the bloodstream, some women (the so-called high-risk women— more about this on page 105) find that they begin to lose bone mass, a condition called osteoporosis. Bones become porous and brittle. This leads to loss of posture—the so-called dowager's hump seen in elderly people. As bone density decreases, there is a greater risk of hip, spine or forearm **fractures**. HRT cannot repair damaged bone, but it has clearly been shown to arrest the progression of osteoporosis.

To protect against heart disease. For years researchers wondered why premenopausal women experienced fewer heart attacks than men of the same age. Today many scientists believe that estrogen is the protective factor. Estrogen is thought to reduce levels of harmful cholesterol (LDL cholesterol) and increase levels of beneficial cholesterol (HDL cholesterol) in the blood, thus giving some measure of protection to women who are susceptible to heart disease.

You may find any of these four potential uses of HRT reason enough to take hormones—particularly if you have a personal or family history of debilitating menopausal symptoms, frequent vaginal or urinary infections, osteoporosis or heart disease. But what if you have no history of these ailments or conditions? For you the decision to take or not take estrogen is less clear-cut.

That's because, for most women, these benefits are not achieved without some adverse effects. These might be minor but bothersome problems such as breast tenderness, migraine headaches, leg cramps, nausea and vomiting. Or HRT's possible adverse effects may be serious, even life-threatening. One form of HRT, known as unopposed estrogen therapy, increases the risk of endometrial cancer two- to fifteenfold. (See "The History of HRT" on the opposite page for a summary of this and other problems with estrogen use.) Several recent studies suggest that estrogen therapy increases the risk of gallstones two- to threefold. But for many the most controversial question about HRT is how it affects a woman's risk of breast cancer. About 40 studies have been done to investigate this question, and researchers still dispute the findings. Some say the data show no connection between HRT and breast cancer; others read into the data an overall increased risk related to dosage and duration of use. For some women, this chance of risk—no matter how small—is enough to make them question the value of HRT.

(continued on page 23)

▌ The History of HRT

Researchers first isolated estrogen and progesterone in the 1920s, and by the 1930s synthetic forms of these hormones were produced for use during menopause. But it wasn't until the 1960s, when researchers understood the use of estrogen and progesterone as **oral contraceptives**, that hormone replacement therapy, in the form of estrogen therapy, became part of the medical arsenal.

The contraceptive pill came on the market first. It was followed by estrogen therapy. In the 1960s and early 1970s, many physicians encouraged their patients to begin daily doses of estrogen long before menopause and continue large doses for life. Estrogen was portrayed as a miracle drug that could keep a woman young forever. This form of HRT made use of a synthetic estrogen called ethinyl estradiol and was given in less-potent doses than oral contraceptives.

Estrogen therapy and contraceptives were not the only uses of estrogen touted by the medical establishment. From the 1940s to the early 1970s, doctors also widely prescribed another synthetic estrogen, diethylstilbestrol (abbreviated as DES), to reduce the risk of miscarriages.

By the 1960s use of the hormone estrogen was fully embraced by the public and the medical profession, and until 1975 menopausal estrogen was one of the most commonly prescribed drugs on this continent. Little thought was given to any long-term side effects of these drugs.

Then in the 1970s, years of accumulated evidence about estrogen's drawbacks were made public. Researchers disclosed that women who had been using the

▼

contraceptive pill since their 20s and 30s faced a much greater risk of heart attack in their 40s, particularly if they were smokers. In 1971 a link was found between the use of DES during pregnancy and a rare form of vaginal cancer; that year the Food and Drug Administration withdrew its approval of DES for use as a pregnancy medication. Evidence continues to show that DES daughters—women exposed to DES before birth—are at higher-than-normal risk for vaginal cancer, while DES mothers have a higher risk for breast cancer.

More evidence about the dangers of estrogen mounted. In 1975 menopausal estrogen therapy was linked to dramatically increased rates of cancer in the uterus—in the range of four to 14 times the norm, depending upon how long a woman had taken the hormone and at what strength.

As these disturbing figures came to light, prescriptions for estrogen therapy plummeted from 1975 to the mid-1980s. The medical world and the pharmaceutical industry scrambled to adjust. DES was removed from the market. Doses of estrogen were reduced for both oral contraceptives and hormone replacement therapy. In addition, researchers developed a new, so-called natural conjugated (combined) estrogen that was collected from animals and more closely matched the chemical composition of human estrogen.

Finally, to address the problem of endometrial cancer, doctors began prescribing **progestin** (a form of progesterone that can be either natural or synthetic) in addition to estrogen. The result was a combined hormone therapy—which today is the mainstay of HRT. They discovered the problem with unopposed estrogen

▼

(estrogen given alone instead of in combination with progestin) was that it stimulated the growth of cells in the uterus. Without progesterone to cause a menstrual period and thus shed those cells, the lining of the uterus (the **endometrium**) became too thick, setting the stage for a slow-growing form of cancer.

As a result of these changes, estrogens have resumed their place in the top 10 pharmaceutical sales hit parade, surpassing sales achieved in the 1960s and 1970s. Today the most commonly prescribed drug in the United States is Premarin, a conjugated estrogen, with some $180 million of it sold each year. Estrogen has made a comeback.

Yes, hormone replacement therapy is big business. But is it good business? Do scientists completely understand the effects, both good and bad, of estrogen on the female body? Or are there further side-effect surprises in store for the American woman in five, 10, 20 years? Only time will tell.

And women aren't the only ones concerned about side effects. Doctors, too, debate the benefits and the risks of hormone replacement, particularly long-term HRT. While some doctors suggest that HRT is suitable for every woman, with very few exceptions, other doctors argue a conservative approach, prescribing HRT only for those at-risk women who have a clear need for the assistance estrogen offers and for whom alternatives to HRT are not appropriate or successful. (See Chapter 6.)

At the heart of these vast differences of opinion is the question: Who will benefit from HRT? This book aims to shed light on every side of the debate.

How HRT Is Used

Hormone replacement therapy, as used in the 1990s, entails taking estrogen and/or progestin in one of several ways:

• **Unopposed estrogen.** This is estrogen given alone. Depending upon the regimen your doctor recommends, the estrogen may be prescribed to be taken for 21 days a month, 25 days a month or without interruption. Generally, unopposed estrogen is prescribed only for women without a uterus; in women with a uterus, unopposed estrogen increases the risk of **hyperplasia** (a proliferation of cells in the uterine lining that can lead to uterine cancer).

In the United States most women take estrogen in one of several pill formulations available by prescription only. The most popular is **conjugated equine estrogen** (sold as Premarin or in generic forms). Derived from the urine of pregnant mares, Premarin is currently used by about 9 million women. The usual daily dose of conjugated estrogen is .625 mg a day.

Other common pill forms of estrogen include **esterified estrogen** (sold as Estratab and Menest) at .625 mg a day, **micronized estradiol** (Estrace) at 1 mg a day, and **estropipate** (Ogen and Ortho-Est) at .625 mg a day. Each of these pill formulations has a slightly different chemical formulation, but they all work in the body in similar ways.

Estrogen comes in other forms—estrogen creams and skin patches are only two of several faces of this drug. (We talk about the alternatives to pills in Chapter 3.)

• **Combination therapy.** In this form of HRT, you take progestin in addition to one of the forms of estrogen mentioned earlier.

Progestin is added for one simple reason: It protects the uterus. You see, constant estrogen stimulation causes the lining of the uterus, the endometrium, to grow and thicken. If it gets too thick, the result is hyperplasia, a condition that can sometimes develop into endometrial cancer. Progestin works to prevent the uterine lining from reaching dangerously thick levels, thus forestalling the risk of endometrial cancer. For that reason most women with a uterus are advised to take progestin along with estrogen. Women who have had a **hysterectomy** do not need progestin.

There are four common estrogen-progestin combination therapy regimens:

- **Cyclic sequential therapy.** In this therapy .625 mg of conjugated estrogen (or an equivalent) is taken for 21 days or 25 days of the month, with 5 to 10 mg a day of progestin taken along with the estrogen for the last 10 or 14 days. Then nothing is taken for five days. Cyclic sequential therapy is designed to mimic the menstrual cycle. During the first few years of using estrogen and cyclic progestin, a woman experiences two or three days of monthly bleeding, followed by light spotting, much like a normal menstrual period.

    The form of progestin generally used is **medroxyprogesterone acetate**, sold as Amen, Cycrin and Provera. Some women receive 2.5 to 5 mg of **norethindrone**, another progestin, if medroxyprogesterone causes premenstrual syndrome-like discomforts.

- **Cyclic combined therapy.** Here the woman takes .625 mg of conjugated estrogen (or an equivalent) and low-dosage progestin (2.5 mg) for 25 days each month, with a five- or six-day rest period. This is a newer form of combination therapy, and preliminary studies of its effectiveness show that there is less unexpected light spotting or bleeding, called **breakthrough bleeding**, compared with continuous combined therapy (see below).

- **Continuous sequential therapy.** Here a woman takes .625 mg of conjugated estrogen (or an equivalent) every day of the month. Progestin (10 mg of medroxyprogesterone or 2.5 to 5 mg of norethindrone or norethindrone acetate) is taken for 12 to 14 days, from the twelfth through the twenty-fifth day of the month. As with the cyclic sequential therapy, there is menstrual-like bleeding at the end of the month.

- **Continuous combined therapy.** In this treatment a small amount of progestin (usually 2.5 mg) and .625 mg of estrogen (or an equivalent) are taken every day of the month. The form of progestin generally used is medroxyprogesterone acetate (Amen, Cycrin and Provera). This therapy is designed to prevent menstrual-like monthly bleeding (which many women dislike) of cyclic sequential and continuous sequential therapies. The trade-off, however, is that women (40 percent after six months) continue to experience up to 20 days of light breakthrough bleeding each month. (We address the subject of breakthrough bleeding and related side effects of hormone replacement therapy in Chapter 3.)

- **Estrogen plus testosterone.** This therapy includes a small dose of **testosterone**, an **androgen** (a steroid hormone that increases growth of male physical qualities). It is sometimes prescribed to women who have had their ovaries and uterus surgically removed and to women in **perimenopause**, the early stages of menopause, and who report a loss of sexual desire. Testosterone increases sexual desire. It can also help relieve breast tenderness, one of the short-term side effects of estrogen therapy, according to Ronald L. Young, M.D., of Baylor College of Medicine in Houston. (We will discuss these side effects in Chapter 3.)

Estratest, an esterified estrogen (1.25 mg a day) with methyltestosterone (1.25 or 2.5 mg a day), and a version of Premarin (.625 mg conjugated estrogen a day) with methyltestosterone are two such drugs on the market.

Is Menopause a Disease?

We've looked at the types of estrogen found naturally in the female body, examined the types of estrogen available in hormone therapy and summarized the types of HRT regimens and what HRT is supposed to achieve. The question remains: Who needs HRT?

As we mentioned early in this chapter, some proponents of HRT assert that every woman is a candidate for HRT. These experts believe women should take estrogen to prevent health problems later in life. Other proponents argue that the treatment is suitable for some, but by no means all, women. Detractors claim that equally positive health effects can be achieved through self-care: sound eating habits, exercise and even alternative therapies. (We'll detail these points in Chapter 6.)

These differences in medical opinion are bewildering. After all, every physician has access to the same research studies and surveys. If you, like we, are trying to understand such varied attitudes toward HRT, you might find it helpful to look at some of the medical establishment's underlying

(continued on page 29)

▎Natural Versus Synthetic

As we've seen, estrogen is actually a collective term, a family name (so to speak) for three related female hormones: estradiol (the most potent and active form), estrone and estriol. These hormones are produced naturally by the body. When health care practitioners talk about hormone replacement, however, they use the word estrogen to describe preparations that are manufactured by pharmaceutical companies. When you take hormone replacement therapy, you are taking estrogen that is similar, but not identical, to human estrogen.

The estrogens prescribed in hormone replacement therapy may be natural or synthetic:

• **Natural estrogens** are called natural because they are naturally occurring and are similar to the estrogens made in the human body. Most hormone replacement therapies call for natural estrogen because it is gentler and closer to human estrogen. Today the most frequently used natural estrogen is Premarin, a conjugated estrogen (which combines five or six types of estrogen) made from the urine of pregnant mares. Other natural estrogens include generic versions of conjugated estrogen, esterified estrogen (Estratab and Menest), micronized (finely ground) estradiol (Estrace), and transdermal estradiol (Estraderm); the latter is applied via the skin.

• **Synthetic estrogens** are synthesized, using petroleum-based chemicals, and are more potent than natural estrogens. They include estropipate (Ogen and Ortho-Est). Stronger synthetic estrogens are used as an active ingredient in birth control pills to stop ovulation.

▼

Hormone replacement therapy usually entails supplementing estrogen with a progesterone, another hormone that is part of a family of hormones known as progestins. Progestins also can be natural or synthetic.

• **Natural progesterone**, as it is generally called, must be made up to order by a pharmacist. Because of this it is not prescribed as often as synthetic progestins, although it has fewer side effects.

• **Synthetic progestins** tend to be more potent than natural progesterones. One synthetic progestin in particular is used routinely in HRT: medroxyprogesterone acetate (Amen, Cycrin, Provera). **Megesterol acetate** (Megace) is sometimes prescribed. Stronger androgenic progestins, such as norethindrone and norgestrel, are primary ingredients in birth control pills.

Which should you use—natural or synthetic? The answer will depend in part on your own health and medical history. Use what you've just learned here as a jumping-off point for a talk with your health care practitioner.

views of menopause. Given the same data, doctors may recommend different ways of "treating" menopause simply because they look at menopause from different perspectives. Here are some of these views of menopause:

Menopause as natural passage. Many physicians see menopause as a natural stage of biological development. These doctors may believe that HRT is unnecessary, or they may believe that HRT is useful for certain women in certain situations—such as women at high risk of osteoporosis or women who have had a hysterectomy at a young age and thus prematurely lost the ability to produce estrogen.

Menopause as disease. Many physicians view menopause as organ failure or a deficiency syndrome and, as such, believe menopause must be medically treated in all or almost all women. A practitioner with this attitude naturally will see HRT as beneficial to all women nearing menopause, because all women are presumed "at risk."

Menopause as unnatural state. Closely related to the view of menopause as disease is the viewpoint that the post-menopausal state is unnatural. According to proponents of this view, the female body was not designed to live many years past menopause. In past centuries, so goes the argument, women rarely lived long past menopause, while in this century women can easily survive 30 years or more in a postmenopausal state, thanks to advancements in health care and nutritional science. This extended life span without estrogen is unnatural, according to this theory, and thus it is unfair to deprive women of HRT and the benefits it can produce. These proponents argue that women should take HRT if they want it.

HRT as natural therapy. This viewpoint asserts that because estrogen is a substance normally produced in a pre-menopausal woman's body, supplementation with estrogen is appropriate, natural and, in most cases, safe.

All these points of view will become clearer as we explore hormone replacement therapy more deeply. But first let's take a look at the female body and the role that hormones play in promoting health.

. . . .

CHAPTER II

Hormones and Your Body

L ong before you began weighing the pros and cons of hormone replacement therapy, your body's hormones were actively at work. Hormones guide every cycle of your body: your growth as a child, your physical transformation from girl to woman, the preparation of your body for childbearing, the gradual cessation of menstruation, the postmenopausal years.

An infant girl is born with all the elements of the female reproductive system. These gradually develop through late childhood and begin functioning as the girl reaches **menarche** (her first menstrual period) sometime between ages 10 and 16. In a similar way the reproductive system slowly stops functioning in midlife as the woman approaches menopause (her last menstrual period) sometime between ages 45 and 55. In between menarche and menopause lie the reproductive years. The entire process of reproductive growth and maturation is controlled by hormones, and the largest role is played by the hormone estrogen. In this chapter we examine estrogen's role in our reproductive function and in our health.

The Female Reproductive System

A woman's reproductive system consists of six major parts: The two ovaries contain the egg follicles that may one day ripen, be fertilized and grow into babies. The two **fallopian tubes** capture eggs as they leave the ovaries and channel them to the uterus **(womb)**, where fertilized eggs may attach to the uterine wall and mature into embryos and then babies. The vagina is the resilient tract by which a baby leaves the womb and enters the world.

The reproductive system is controlled by the actions of many interrelated organs or glands, which secrete complex chemicals known as hormones, thereby producing effects in other parts of the body. Technically known as the **endocrine system**, this network of glands manufactures hormones and releases them into the bloodstream. Hormones act as chemical messengers. They travel via the blood to specific organs (sometimes called target organs), where they exert their effect. The body has many hormone-producing glands: The stomach, for instance, produces gastrin, a hormone that stimulates the production of food-dissolving juices. The islets of Langerhans in the pancreas produce insulin, a hormone that enables the body to convert sweet and starchy foods into energy to power the body.

In women the reproductive part of the endocrine system is overseen by the **hypothalamus**, a small but powerful gland in the brain. The hypothalamus works in conjunction with the **pituitary** (a pebble-sized gland beneath the hypothalamus) and the ovaries (two almond-shaped glands alongside the uterus that contain unfertilized egg cells) to regulate the menstrual cycle throughout childbearing years.

These four organs (the hypothalamus, the pituitary and the two ovaries) are also responsible for starting the process that transforms a girl into a woman.

The Prepubescent and Pubescent Years

In the first eight years of life, hormones encourage a child to grow in physical size, physical strength and mental capacity. In these early years, the hormone estrogen is produced in tiny amounts in the female body. The male hormone testosterone also makes up a tiny proportion of hormones in a girl's body, but by the time she reaches age nine or 10, her body produces more estrogen than testosterone.

Between ages nine and 14, the pituitary gland in a girl's brain begins producing a hormone known as **follicle-stimulating hormone (FSH)**, which stimulates the ovaries to start their production of estrogen. With new, higher levels of estrogen circulating through the bloodstream, a girl's body gains adult female characteristics. Breasts develop; pubic and underarm hair appears. Inside the body, the vagina, uterus, fallopian tubes and ovaries increase in size. This period is known as **puberty**.

Finally, menstruation begins, usually around ages 12 to 14 (although it can begin as early as age nine and as late as age 16). Pregnancy becomes possible.

In the first one to three years after menarche, a young woman's body continues to mature. Her hips broaden, she stops growing in height and her menstrual periods—often irregular at first—become regular and of predictable duration (usually around 28 days in length). These changes are all due to the presence of the hormone estrogen in her body.

The Reproductive Years

From the time a woman's menstrual cycle becomes regular until her childbearing years end (generally somewhere between ages 45 and 55), her body is on a monthly cycle of hormone release and response.

Every month the hypothalamus produces and sends **gonadotropin-releasing hormones** (also called releasing factors) to the pituitary gland. The pituitary in turn manufactures two hormones called **gonadotropins**. In the first few days of the menstrual cycle, the pituitary gland secretes the gonadotropin FSH (the same follicle-stimulating hormone that caused a girl's ovaries to begin producing estrogen). FSH awakens several dormant egg cells in one of the ovaries and directs those cells to ripen. As the eggs grow, they produce estradiol, a form of estrogen. The estradiol enters the bloodstream and helps thicken the lining of uterus to receive a fertilized egg.

About two weeks into the menstrual cycle, one egg follicle dominates and protrudes from the surface of the ovary. Estradiol levels in the bloodstream peak. The hypothalamus then sends another message to the pituitary gland to stop producing FSH and begin manufacturing the gonadotropin **luteinizing hormone (LH)**. LH causes the ripe egg to burst from its follicle on the ovary, an event known as ovulation. The egg falls into one of the fallopian tubes—two narrow structures that catch the egg at ovulation, provide a place for sperm to fertilize the egg and propel the egg to the uterus.

For several days the ruptured follicle's scar tissue acts as another **endocrine gland**. Known as the **corpus luteum**, this temporary gland manufactures the female hormone progesterone. The progesterone relaxes the uterine muscles, prepares the endometrium (uterine lining) to accept a fertilized egg and causes the uterine walls to form blood vessels and stockpile the nutrients that can support a fetus.

If the egg is not fertilized, the progesterone breaks down the thickened, blood-enriched lining of the uterus. Sloughed-off blood and unneeded cells are shed from the body in the process known as menstruation (the menstrual period). Menstruation occurs during the final week of the menstrual cycle and lasts an average of three to five days. Then the whole process begins again.

▌ Other Hormones to Know

Estrogen and progesterone are the best-known hormones in the female reproductive cycle. Estrogen starts the transition from childhood to puberty, and estrogen helps thicken the lining of the uterus to receive a fertilized egg. Progesterone helps the uterus develop the structure to support a fertilized egg and, if the egg is not fertilized, progesterone causes menstruation.

But other hormones affect your body's growth, as well as the long-term health of your body after menopause, and thus tie into this book's discussions of HRT. So make your acquaintance with this cast of characters:

The **adrenal glands**, located alongside the kidneys, produce several hormones: mineralocorticoids, which, among other jobs, maintain the balance of salt and fluids in the body; glucocorticoids, which help regulate blood sugar and blood pressure and help the body avoid fatigue; testosterone, a male sex hormone found in small

▼

amounts in women; and epinephrine (adrenaline) and norepinephrine, the so-called stress hormones. The adrenal glands also produce the hormone **androstenedione**, which fatty tissue in the body converts into estrone, a form of estrogen.

The **thyroid gland**, located in the throat just below the larynx, or voice box, secretes three hormones. Two of these, T_3 (short for triiodothyronine) and T_4 (thyroxine), affect how well cells consume oxygen, thus affecting the growth and development of every part of the body. The third thyroid hormone, **calcitonin**, decreases calcium in the bloodstream and is thought to help bones absorb calcium. (We'll discuss calcitonin again in Chapter 6.)

The **parathyroids**, four small glands attached alongside the thyroid, manufacture **parathyroid hormone**, which acts to maintain an even amount of calcium in the blood.

Hormones are often assisted by hormone-like fatty acids (sometimes called **mediators**) produced in tiny amounts in body tissues such as the uterus. If hormones are the chemical messengers, the mediators are the chemicals that actually carry out the job. One such mediator, **prostaglandin**, causes contractions in the uterus during menstruation and during the labor phase of pregnancy. It also affects blood pressure. Another body chemical, **cyclic AMP (cAMP)**, is involved in nervous system, hormone and cell functions.

Remember these characters in the hormone replacement story. Because the body's endocrine system is closely interwoven, all these hormones interact with estrogen and progesterone and play a role in long-term health both before and after menopause.

Hormonal Birth Control

Although the hormones estrogen and progesterone are usually plentiful in the female body during the reproductive years, many premenopausal women take additional amounts of these hormones as a method of birth control. In fact, you probably first became acquainted with hormone use through conversations with friends and physicians about birth control.

The birth control pill (otherwise known as the oral contraceptive or **the Pill**) has been on the market since the 1960s. Taken daily and usually made of a combination of estrogen and progestin (a usually synthetic form of progesterone), the oral contraceptive suppresses ovulation; makes the cervical mucus thick and sticky so that sperm cannot enter the uterus; and prevents the uterine wall from thickening, thus reducing the chance that a fertilized egg can grow. In general oral contraceptives are 98 percent effective, meaning that two out of every 100 women using them will become pregnant. Usually this is because they have missed a pill.

Yesteryear's oral contraceptives contained high doses of estrogen (up to 150 **micrograms** [mcg, one-millionth of a gram] a day) and progestin (up to 10 mg a day) and were associated with serious side effects such as blood clots leading to heart attack and stroke, gallbladder disease, noncancerous liver tumors and high blood pressure.

Today's birth control pills come in significantly lower doses—up to 35 mcg of estrogen and from .15 to 2.5 mg of progestin a day. They are as effective in preventing pregnancy as their forebears. But are these newer contraceptives safer? The answer is not clear because few long-term studies of the effects of newer, lower-dose contraceptives have been completed. However, some short-term studies suggest that the cardiovascular risks have decreased with the newer contraceptives, according to Beverly Winikoff, M.D., and her colleagues in *The Contraceptive Handbook: A Guide to Safe and Effective Choices*. Common, less serious side effects such as breast swelling and nausea appear to be less common among women using the newer Pill, she adds.

If you smoke, you should not use oral contraceptives, no matter what your age, Winikoff writes. In women who smoke, the risk of heart attack increases twelvefold, she says; in women who smoke and take oral contraceptives, the risk of heart attack increases fiftyfold.

Based on what is known about the safety of oral contraceptives to date, the writers of *The Contraceptive Handbook* state that you should NOT take oral contraceptives: if you are pregnant; if you have a history of blood clots in the lungs, eyes or deep veins of the legs (this does not include varicose veins or hemorrhoids); if you have a history of **angina** (chest pain cause by insufficient blood flow to the heart); if you have cancer of the breast, cervix, vagina or uterus; if you smoke; if you were diagnosed with jaundice during pregnancy or an earlier use of oral contraceptives; or if you have any undiagnosed abnormal vaginal bleeding.

Further, some medical conditions are associated with the more severe side effects of oral contraceptives. Therefore, women with the following conditions should check with their doctors before using the Pill: high blood pressure, heart disease, family history of early heart attack or stroke, elevated cholesterol or triglycerides (blood fats), kidney disease, gallbladder disease, severe migraine headaches, epilepsy, severe diabetes and severe mental depression.

Other less serious side effects of oral contraceptives include acne or unsightly hair growth, weight gain, depression, fluid retention, nervousness, irritability, headache, decreased sexual desire, fatigue and bloating. Oral contraceptives may also prevent the intestines from absorbing important vitamins and minerals, says Howard I. Shapiro, M.D., in *The New Birth Control Book*. These nutrients include vitamins B_1 (thiamine), B_2 (riboflavin), B_6 (pyridoxine), B_{11} (folic acid) and B_{12} (cobalamin), vitamin C (ascorbic acid), vitamin E (alphatocopherol) and zinc. Most studies attempting to link oral contraceptives and cancer have been negative.

Despite the apparent drawbacks of oral contraceptive use, birth control pills offer some health benefits beyond preventing unwanted pregnancies, according to Morris Notelovitz, M.D., author of *Menopause and Midlife Health*. Women using estrogen-containing oral contraceptives are 70 percent less likely to develop benign (harmless or nonmalignant) ovarian cysts and 40 percent less likely to develop ovarian cancer than nonusers, he says. They are less likely to develop benign breast cysts, to develop iron-deficiency anemia or to contract **pelvic inflammatory disease** (a serious bacterial infection of the uterus, fallopian tubes and/or ovaries). Studies suggest that estrogen-containing oral contraceptives offer some protection against endometrial cancer and increase **bone mass** about 1 percent per year, Notelovitz adds.

What's Available in Birth Control Pills

Oral contraceptives all contain synthetic (man-made) hormones—usually an estrogen (mestranol or ethinyl estradiol are the two synthetic estrogens used in birth control) plus one of six different progestins: ethynodiol diacetate, levonorgestrel, norethindrone, norethindrone acetate, norgestrel and norethynodrel. Oral contraceptives come in four types—the first three are combination pills of estrogen and progestin:

• **Single-phase**, or **monophasic**, **pills** contain the same amount of estrogen and progestin in each pill throughout the cycle. These pills contain a higher total amount of hormones than other types.

• **Biphasic pills** contain a steady dose of estrogen (35 mcg) throughout the cycle. The first 10 pills (for the first 10 days) also contain .05 mg of progestin; the last 11 pills contain 1 mg of progestin. The change in progestin levels is an attempt to mimic the menstrual cycle. Biphasic pills are not very popular because women often experience unexpected bleeding between menstrual periods—called breakthrough bleeding.

• **Triphasic pills** vary the amount of both estrogen and progestin during the month. Again the idea is to mimic the menstrual cycle. Triphasic pills must be taken in the proper sequence throughout the month, making these contraceptives more of a challenge to use correctly. However, they have a lower total amount of hormones than their single-phase and biphasic cousins.

• **Progestin-only pills**, dubbed "minipills," contain small amounts of progestin (.075 mg of norgestrel or .35 mg of norethindrone) and no estrogen at all. They are taken every day of the month and are less forgiving of changes in timing (they must be taken at the same time each day), dosage and consistency in taking the pill. It has a slightly higher failure rate than the phasic contraceptives, in part because it does not always prevent ovulation. Of 100 women using the minipill in any one year, two to eight of them will become pregnant.

(continued on page 42)

▌Birth Control and Hormone Replacement: What's the Difference?

What are the differences between birth control pills and hormone replacement therapy? The most obvious difference is who uses them. Birth control pills, or oral contraceptives as they're also called, are used by women before menopause. Hormone replacement therapy is used by women during and after menopause.

Oral contraceptives contain much higher doses of estrogen and progestin than HRT. Oral contraceptives exclusively use synthetic estrogen and progestin, which are stronger than their natural counterparts. These higher doses of estrogen and progestin are needed in contraceptives to prevent ovulation and/or fertilization of eggs.

High doses of estrogen and progestin, however, are not needed to relieve menopause-related hot flashes or protect against osteoporosis, so today's hormone replacement regimens contain smaller amounts of hormones than birth control pills. In addition, most women using HRT today are prescribed the milder, "natural" conjugated estrogen Premarin, which is derived from animal urine and more closely matches human estrogen than the synthetic estrogens devised in a laboratory setting. Although most women use a synthetic progesterone in their HRT regimen, a natural progesterone is available.

The progestin-only pills pose different health risks than phasic contraceptives. Possible increased risks from the minipill include ovarian cysts, **ectopic pregnancy** (in which a fertilized egg implants itself in a fallopian tube instead of the uterus) and erratic bleeding (breakthrough bleeding, long menstrual periods, more frequent menstrual periods or no periods at all).

Premature Menopause and Hormone Replacement

Although most women do not need hormone replacement during their reproductive years, about 9 percent of women experience menopause before age 40. This situation is known as a **premature menopause**, and it is the number one reason young women find themselves candidates for hormone replacement therapy.

What provokes premature menopause? In some cases, there are no precise answers. But there are common causes or factors for this rare situation:

Surgical removal of the ovaries (called **oophorectomy**) is the most frequent cause of an early menopause. Oophorectomies are usually done along with a hysterectomy, or removal of the uterus. Without ovaries, your body no longer produces estradiol, the body's major source of estrogen in the reproductive years, and menopause immediately begins.

Menopause caused by surgical removal of the ovaries is aptly called **surgical menopause** or **artificial menopause**. Estimates are that 25 percent of women in the United States reach menopause by means of removal of their ovaries.

If your ovaries are still producing estradiol (and they probably are if you are under 45) at the time they are surgically removed, then you will probably experience dramatic or severe menopausal symptoms such as hot flashes. These menopause-related discomforts are often more severe than those that accompany a natural, nonsurgical menopause because of the suddenness of the removal of the ovaries, writes Wulf H. Utian, M.D., in *Managing Your Menopause*. Doctors today relate the severity of menopause discomforts to the abruptness of estradiol decline. As a rule, the more abrupt the drop in estrogen levels, the more intense the symptoms of menopause. Surgical removal of the ovaries causes estrogen levels to plummet. (We will explain this further in Chapter 3.)

According to the National Center for Health Statistics, 562,000 hysterectomies were performed in 1993. Of those, 326,000 were performed on women ages 15 to 44. At the time of surgery to remove the uterus, many doctors recommend that the ovaries also be removed, even if they are healthy, because of the risk that the woman may develop ovarian cancer.

Ovarian cancer accounts for 5 percent of all cancers diagnosed among women. The risk for ovarian cancer increases with a woman's age. It is seldom seen in women under age 35. The average age of a woman diagnosed with ovarian cancer is 60, but many women are not diagnosed with the disease until 75 or 80. Studies show that the actual risk of developing ovarian cancer after the uterus is removed is much lower. Only 6 percent of ovarian cancers develop in ovaries that were left behind after a hysterectomy, according to the medical textbook *Current Obstetric and Gynecologic Diagnosis and Treatment*.

In women under 40, **prophylactic** (that is, preventive) removal of the ovaries in women who are undergoing hysterectomy for noncancerous conditions "is of questionable value," the authors of *Current Obstetric and Gynecologic Diagnosis and Treatment* write.

The major reason that ovary removal is questionable is the fact that your ovaries produce large amounts of estradiol during your reproductive years and smaller, but equally valuable, amounts of other estrogens for 10, 15, 20 years after menopause. Medical science is only beginning to understand how valuable these non-estradiol estrogens can be in the postmenopausal years. If you are a candidate for the removal of your uterus, you and your medical practitioner must weigh the benefits of retaining healthy ovaries against the risk of ovarian cancer.

Smoking can bring on early menopause. Doctors are not sure why this happens. Wulf Utian in *Managing Your Menopause* points to two current theories: that some substance in cigarette smoke causes estrogen's destruction, or that the nicotine in cigarette smoke reduces the blood supply to the ovary and causes it to fail prematurely.

Radiation therapy to treat pelvic cancer destroys the ovaries. Chemical therapy (chemotherapy) to treat other cancers, such as breast cancer, can sometimes (but not always) destroy the egg follicles or the ovaries.

Other theories for early menopause include the presence of an autoimmune disorder (in which the body produces antibodies that disturb the ovaries or destroy ovarian tissue) or the role of genetics. If your mother had an early menopause, you are likely to have an early menopause too. It may be that some women are born with fewer egg follicles or that they have some condition that causes the body to stop producing estrogen while they are still young.

If you have an early menopause, should you take hormone replacement therapy? The medical literature suggests that long-term estrogen deprivation, whatever its cause, puts you at a greater risk of developing osteoporosis and cardiovascular disease later in your life. The younger you are at menopause, the sooner you are exposed to the long-term consequences of estrogen deficiency. (We'll discuss these issues in Chapter 5.)

Most mainstream medical practitioners recommend that women who have experienced premature menopause begin HRT. And apparently many women follow this advice, particularly those who have their ovaries surgically removed. A study of patterns of estrogen use found that women who had surgical menopause (the number one cause of premature menopause) were 10 times more likely to take HRT than women who had a natural menopause (*American Journal of Epidemiology*, September 1, 1994).

Is there a special HRT regimen for women who have had an early menopause? No. As long as you have no medical conditions that prohibit your using HRT, you have a choice of the full range of treatment options. (We address these medical conditions and treatment regimens in Chapter 3.) If you cannot use HRT or choose not to, you may wish to follow some of the alternative therapies described in Chapter 6.

■ Oophorectomies and Hysterectomies— Are They Necessary?

Doctors who perform oophorectomies—surgical removal of the ovaries—expose women to more years of hormone replacement if those women elect to take hormone replacement therapy. Why remove ovaries in the first place? Both ovaries may be removed because they have been rendered nonfunctional by ovarian tumors, pelvic inflammatory disease, **endometriosis** or cancer.

But all too often in the United States, doctors recommend that a woman over age 40 who is having a hysterectomy should also have her ovaries removed, on the grounds that she may develop ovarian cancer later in life. These doctors reason that a woman over 40 is probably only a few years away from menopause anyhow, so why not remove the soon-to-be-useless ovaries and reduce the risk of cancer?

There are several flaws in this argument. For one, the actual risk of developing ovarian cancer after the uterus is removed is low: Only 6 percent of ovarian cancers develop in ovaries that were left behind after a hysterectomy, according to *Current Obstetric and Gynecologic Diagnosis and Treatment*. For another, most women don't go through menopause until age 45 to 55, and until then their ovaries continue to pump out estrogen. In light of the protective effect of estrogen on bone health and heart disease and the **atrophic** changes that occur when estrogen levels fall, it doesn't seem prudent to remove the natural source of estrogen—the ovaries—from

▼

women who are otherwise healthy, especially since those very same doctors will turn around and recommend hormone replacement to those women whose ovaries are gone.

Fewer ovaries would be removed if fewer hysterectomies were performed. Research has shown that 30 to 50 percent of the hysterectomies in the United States are clearly unnecessary; another 10 percent could be avoided if women were offered other therapies, according to the Boston Women's Health Book Collective book *The New Our Bodies, Ourselves.* In about 40 percent of hysterectomies, the ovaries are also removed.

Hysterectomies are most likely to be performed for **fibroid** tumors, uterine prolapse or endometriosis. This doesn't mean that the operation is your best choice for any one of these conditions, however. All three can be treated by other means—and usually it's a good idea to get a second opinion from a doctor specializing in your particular condition to see if you have alternatives to surgery.

A hysterectomy *is* necessary for cancer of the uterus, vagina, fallopian tubes or ovaries and usually for invasive cervical cancer; for severe uncontrollable infection (usually associated with pelvic inflammatory disease); for severe, uncontrollable bleeding; for life-threatening blockages of the bladder or bowels by the uterus or growths on the uterus; and for rare complications of childbirth, such as uterine rupture.

The Perimenopausal Years

Perimenopause refers to the years immediately before menopause. Most women enter perimenopause by their late 40s. Since natural menopause, however, can occur by age 45, some women enter perimenopause by their late 30s.

The exact age varies from woman to woman. But for most of us, somewhere from two to six years before our last menstrual period our ovaries have difficulty producing viable egg follicles. It's not that we necessarily run out of eggs, as is commonly said; it's that ovarian function declines. The ovaries simply fail to respond to the command "ripen an egg" delivered by the follicle-stimulating hormone produced by the pituitary gland in the brain. The ovaries release eggs irregularly instead of monthly. Eventually no more egg follicles ripen, and the body stops ovulating.

During this time your ovaries continue to produce estrogen partly out of habit and partly in a final attempt to keep the reproductive process going. In contrast, production of the second important female hormone, progesterone, becomes erratic. Progesterone, as you recall, is manufactured immediately after ovulation by a ruptured egg follicle's scar tissue, and it causes your body to shed the thickened, blood-enriched lining of the uterus in the process known as menstruation. So while the estrogen in your body continues to build up the endometrium (uterine lining) to accept a fertilized egg, menstruation can only occur if progesterone is present. When ovulation becomes irregular, your body does not have the progesterone to cause regular menstrual periods.

Thus, during the perimenopausal years, menstrual periods become unpredictable. Usually they become less frequent, although some women have more frequent periods just before menopause. Menstrual periods disappear for several months and then reappear. They may become heavier or lighter in flow than you have been used to, and the duration of these periods may be shorter or longer than in the past. For most women menstrual-cycle changes are the first flag of the approach of menopause.

Be aware that, as a perimenopausal woman, you are technically still in your reproductive years. Although menstrual periods may be irregular, your body is still releasing eggs and pregnancy is possible.

The irregular menstrual cycles may last only a few months or may continue for four or five years before menstruation ultimately ceases. A few women experience no menstrual irregularities at all. Up to 20 percent of perimenopausal women experience the discomforts associated with menopause itself, particularly hot flashes and vaginal dryness.

Irregular and unusually heavy or light bleeding may be signs of pregnancy or other health problems, so it's wise to talk to your health care practitioner when your menstrual periods become erratic or unusual. One danger in the perimenopausal years is that you may develop hyperplasia (a proliferation of cells). Because there's enough estrogen being produced to build up the endometrium and insufficient progesterone to cause a regular or thorough bleed, your endometrium may become thicker than normal. Eventually the cells proliferate and become so thick that hyperplasia develops.

▮ Medical Tests During Perimenopause

If you are in your 30s or 40s and are having menstrual irregularities, your doctor may suspect that you are entering your perimenopausal years. To confirm this, your physician may want to perform one or more of these medical tests and procedures:

• **FSH test.** Physicians use this blood test to determine whether a woman is approaching or has reached menopause. The test measures the amount of follicle-stimulating hormone (FSH)—the hormone that tells dormant egg cells in the ovaries to ripen. This hormone is circulating in the bloodstream. As you near menopause, your ovaries respond more slowly to FSH, so the pituitary gland in the brain works overtime to make more of this hormone. Levels of FSH in the bloodstream rise.

In a premenopausal woman FSH levels are lower than 30 **international units** per milliliter of blood (abbreviated as 30 IU/ml or as 30 MIU/ml). Levels greater than 30 IU/ml indicate that you are perimenopausal and menopause is imminent, even if you are having menstrual periods.

Eventually your levels of FSH pass the 40 IU/ml mark—sometimes nearing 1,000. Once they have reached 40 IU/ml, FSH levels rarely fall below that measurement. Thus, the 40 IU/ml mark is one sign of the onset of menopause; another is the cessation of menstrual periods.

For the most accurate reading, the FSH test should not be done at mid-menstrual cycle, as FSH levels are normally higher during ovulation.

• **Progesterone challenge test.** This test determines if irregular periods are caused by insufficient proges-

▼

terone. It can be used alone or to confirm the results of a FSH test.

In this test you take progestin (a synthetic or natural form of progesterone) for one week a month for several months. If the progestin makes menstrual periods regular and normal in flow, then you probably have entered perimenopause.

• **Endometrial biopsy.** This is an in-office procedure in which the physician takes a small sample of your endometrium (uterine lining). The sample is examined under a microscope, measured for thickness and analyzed for the presence of abnormal cells.

Endometrial biopsies are one way to check out irregular bleeding and make sure it is not due to hyperplasia (a proliferation of cells in the endometrium that can set the stage for cancer) or another health condition.

Hormones During the Perimenopausal Years

Is hormone therapy needed during the perimenopausal years? Could—or should—a perimenopausal woman start HRT to smooth the transition to menopause? There are two hormone regimens associated with perimenopause; let's examine them:

Progestin alone. To combat irregular and erratic periods, your doctor may prescribe a regimen of progestin only, usually taken in doses of 10 mg a day for seven days. The week's worth of progestin will cause you to menstruate each month until your estrogen levels become too low. (This regimen is just like the progesterone challenge test discussed previously.) Your periods will eventually stop, even if you take progestin. When your body no longer produces enough estrogen to cause the uterine lining to thicken every month, you have entered menopause.

You would continue this therapy for several months at your doctor's direction. A progestin regimen helps prevent that abnormally heavy accumulation of tissue in the uterine lining known as hyperplasia.

Progestin therapy is not without side effects. In many women it causes fluid retention, mood changes and cramps. (Chapter 3 takes a closer look at the side effects of taking progestin, either with or without estrogen.)

Estrogen and progestin. Taking estrogen in combination with progestin (HRT) during perimenopause was once advocated as a way to fend off the discomforts of menopause. Today, however, fewer doctors recommend HRT for women who are still menstruating. The argument is that if you are producing enough estrogen to thicken the endometrium, then you don't need hormone supplements to ease you into menopause or to protect against the long-term complications (osteoporosis, cardiovascular disease and chronic vaginal dryness and irritation) of estrogen deficiency that we highlighted in Chapter 1.

Lila Nachtigall, M.D., writing in *Estrogen: The Facts Can Change Your Life,* explains that during perimenopause your body occasionally generates extremely high levels of estrogen in response to the high level of follicle-stimulating hormone in the bloodstream. FSH, you remember, is high because the pituitary gland is trying to ripen dormant eggs in the now-sluggish ovary. Adding more estrogen to your body by taking HRT can send the already skyrocketing estrogen levels into orbit. Combine this high estrogen level with the low progesterone level that develops when you are not ovulating regularly, and the lining of the endometrium could rapidly proliferate and thicken, setting the stage for hyperplasia or endometrial cancer.

Having said that, Nachtigall acknowledges that there are rare cases in which a perimenopausal woman can begin estrogen therapy: when she is still having periods but suffering from frequent and severe hot flashes and other menopausal discomforts. In such rare cases, Nachtigall says, a physician may prescribe a brief course of HRT (less than six months) as long as a vaginal biopsy is first taken.

During this biopsy the doctor removes a small tissue sample from the walls of the vagina. The sample is examined under a microscope for the presence of a type of cell called **cornified**. Cornified cells develop on the surface of the vagina after estrogen levels have been depleted for several months or more. Their presence indicates that the woman is producing very little estrogen, and Nachtigall feels that it would be safe for her to take estrogen therapy (provided the woman has no health conditions that bar her use of HRT).

Is HRT necessary if you are a perimenopausal women with severe menopausal symptoms? No, it can be a choice. But there are other ways to deal with the discomforts associated with the menopausal years, including other medications, nutritional approaches and self-help strategies (see Chapter 6). If you and your physician are thinking about beginning HRT during your perimenopause, you should learn more about who should not take HRT and what you should expect from the pre-HRT physical examination. We provide this information in Chapter 3.

The Menopausal Years

Technically speaking, *menopause* is a medical term that signifies the normal and complete cessation of menstrual cycles, including both ovulation and menstrual periods. In this usage menopause is a single point in time, a discrete event—your last menstrual period.

In real life it's easy to be confused about where you sit on the medical time line between your reproductive, your perimenopausal or your menopausal years. And that's understandable. If you have gone six months without having a period, how are you to know whether you are perimenopausal or menopausal?

The presence of menopausal symptoms (hot flashes, night sweats, insomnia) can suggest that you are beyond the perimenopausal stage. But as we saw just a few paragraphs ago, some perimenopausal women can have menopausal discomforts. A doctor can confirm that you have entered menopause if:

• *You are over age 40 and have gone 12 consecutive months without a menstrual period,* or

• *Your follicle-stimulating hormone test shows FSH levels above 40 IU/ml.*

Even if your FSH levels are high, by the way, many doctors recommend that you wait till 12 months after your last period before giving up birth control, unless you are trying to conceive. Nature has a way of making your last ovulations completely unpredictable ones.

What causes the female body to cross the (admittedly scientific) boundary from perimenopause to menopause? Here's a quick look at what happens in the body at this stage of the climacteric.

The Changes at Menopause

As we discussed in the section on perimenopause, shorter or irregular periods are the first signals of change in hormones leading to the transition from regular menstrual cycles to menopause.

At menopause blood levels of estradiol, one of the three forms of estrogen, begin to decrease. Estradiol is produced by ripening egg follicles; when your ovaries quit ripening eggs, estradiol isn't formed. Levels of FSH, the follicle-stimulating hormone (which awakens dormant eggs), and LH, the luteinizing hormone (which encourages the ripe egg to burst from the ovary), both skyrocket as the pituitary gland tries to keep the reproductive cycle going.

This joint effort of the FSH and LH works for a while in perimenopause. But one day the FSH and LH no longer have any effect on the ovaries. Sheldon H. Cherry, M.D., and Carolyn D. Runowicz, M.D., authors of *The Menopause Book,* call this situation "ovarian shutdown," and they say it's the cause of menopause itself. Once out of business, the ovaries cease production of estradiol.

In response to the fall in estrogen levels, atrophic (degenerative) changes begin to affect the female body. Estrogen-sensitive organs get smaller and estrogen-sensitive tissues waste away: The ovaries and the uterus shrink. The breasts lose layers of fat and glandular tissue. The endometrium, no longer needed to receive a fertilized egg, thins. The vaginal walls, no longer needed as a birth canal, become thinner and less elastic. The tissues of the **urethra** become thin. Even bone mass begins to decrease. In effect the physical growth and development that estrogen spurred and nurtured in adolescence are now reversed.

These changes affect women to varying degrees. Some women, for example, will notice dry and easily irritated vaginal walls just a few months after menopause; others will never experience any noticeable change in vaginal health.

One reason for the woman-to-woman variation in the amount of atrophic change has to do with the amount of estrogen that the body continues to produce. While the ovaries, a woman's major source of estradiol, drastically curtail estrogen production at menopause, other tissues appear to pick up some of the estrogen slack. For instance, fat cells convert a hormone called androstenedione, pro-duced by the adrenal glands, into the form of estrogen known as estrone. Women with lots of body fat produce more estrone than thin women. The continued presence of estrogen—although not at the same levels as in premeno-pausal years—after menopause may be one reason some women experience fewer atrophic changes than their peers, particularly the loss of bone mass related to osteoporosis. (Look for a discussion of osteoporosis in Chapter 4.)

Atrophic changes take years to develop—if they develop at all. In contrast, menopausal discomforts (such as hot flashes, palpitations, insomnia and night sweats) can occur the moment that estradiol levels in the blood plummet. These discomforts are a sign of the hormonal upheaval your body is going through. As the body gets accustomed to its new estrogen levels (usually within two to five years), menopausal discomforts fade away.

Hormone replacement therapy is often offered as a med-ical treatment to alleviate these short-term discomforts and to slow or prevent atrophic changes to estrogen-sensitive tissues. The role of estrogen and hormone replacement therapy in menopause is the subject of the next chapter.

CHAPTER III

HRT and the Treatment of Menopausal Symptoms

Around 25 percent of women glide through menopause, noticing the cessation of their menstrual periods but experiencing few stresses or discomforts. The remaining 75 percent—most of us—feel the effects of decreased estrogen levels in the form of hot flashes, sleepless nights, strange skin sensations, palpitations or mood swings—the so-called classic complaints of menopause. These signs may be fleeting, manageable or intolerable. No one can predict how you will fare at this time of life.

If you are part of the lucky 25 percent of women who have a stress-free menopause, you and your doctor may give little heed to hormone replacement therapy. But if your menopause symptoms are disruptive or intolerable, interfering with sleep and lifestyle, then you and your doctor may consider hormone replacement therapy. More than 11 million women over age 45 use HRT annually.

The point to remember is that HRT use at menopause is by no means a given, nor is HRT the only way to treat menopausal symptoms. (We cover alternative approaches in Chapter 6.) You may not need hormones; you may not want them. You may decide to take HRT for a short time—one to five years—just to ease through the worst of your hot flashes. Or you may decide to take HRT for 10, 20, 30 years as possible protection against heart disease or osteoporosis later in life. (We discuss this aspect of hormone use in Chapter 4.) Whatever you decide, make it an educated decision.

What Are the Common Menopausal Symptoms?

In medical parlance there are two common types of menopausal symptoms: **vasomotor symptoms** and **genitourinary symptoms**.

Vasomotor Symptoms

Vasomotor symptoms are those that relate to the nerves and muscles that open and close blood vessels. Vasomotor problems generally disappear within five years after menopause, although sometimes they last longer. They include:

• **Hot flashes.** These are the most common vasomotor symptom—as well as the most common and characteristic complaint of menopause. Otherwise known as a **hot flush**, a hot flash is a sensation of intense warmth and a pink flush in the head, neck and upper body. A hot flash can last from a few seconds to two minutes. Some women say their flashes last up to an hour. Typically the hot flash is accompanied by heavy perspiration and rapid pulse and followed by chills and shivering.

Seventy-five percent of women feel hot flashes at some

time during their menopause. Hot flashes can be mild or intense; a daily, fleeting sensation of warmth or a series (up to 50 a day) of sweats and chills that disrupts sleep and leads to exhaustion and irritability. While most women's hot flashes disappear within five years of menopause, approximately 25 percent of women experience hot flashes for six to 10 years and 10 percent have hot flashes 10 years after their last period.

What causes hot flashes? Current thought is that they are related to two things. The first is the abrupt drop in ovarian estrogen (estradiol) that occurs once you enter menopause. The key word here is *abrupt*. Scientists hypothesize that flashes are due to sudden drops in estradiol levels rather than low levels of estradiol in general. It's for this reason scientists suspect that women who have had surgical menopause (both ovaries were surgically removed) tend to have the most severe hot flashes for years after menopause.

The second cause of hot flashes appears to be a disruption of your body's master thermostat (part of the hypothalamus gland in your brain) by gonadotropins (hormones). Here's how the thermostat usually works: When your body temperature is high—perhaps because you have a fever or you've been exercising vigorously—the hypothalamus releases signals that tell the body to dilate (widen) blood vessels, so that more blood travels to the skin and transfers excess heat. High temperatures also alert the hypothalamus to activate the sweat glands under the skin, also cooling your body. When your body temperature is low—perhaps you've been outdoors in cold weather—the hypothalamus tells the blood vessels to constrict (narrow) to reduce heat loss. The gland also tells your body to produce heat through shivering.

During menopause this thermostat may go awry, acting as though your body temperature has increased (when in fact it has not), thus causing the body to start the cool-down process by transferring excess heat to the skin and activating the sweat glands. Hot flashes and drenching sweats are the result. During a hot flash, skin temperature can increase anywhere from 8 to 12 degrees.

How well does HRT remedy hot flashes? "Estrogens are remarkably effective in eliminating this annoying symptom," says Wulf H. Utian, M.D., in *Managing Your Menopause*. In fact, the consensus in the medical community is that estrogen decreases the frequency and severity of hot flashes and other vasomotor symptoms better than any other product on the market. Estrogens not only block the physiologic changes that cause hot flashes, they also enhance the hypothalamus gland's production of natural **opiates**—chemicals that cause sleep or help ease pain.

How many women see relief from hot flashes with HRT? Quite a few, apparently. "Estrogen therapy ameliorates these vasomotor symptoms in the majority of cases," write Bruce R. Carr, M.D., and Jean D. Wilson, M.D., in *Harrison's Principles of Internal Medicine*. Your doctor will expect to see a marked improvement two weeks to two months after you start the therapy.

Hot flashes are not the only vasomotor symptom that have been attributed to the sudden drop in estrogen which occurs at the time of menopause. Other vasomotor symptoms include:

• **Sleep problems.** Such problems—for instance, insomnia—are often caused by hot flashes. Women with frequent hot flashes may be awakened hourly because they feel so warm and/or sweaty. Over the course of days and months, such disrupted sleep can cause memory lapses and feelings of anxiety, according to *Current Obstetric and Gynecologic Diagnosis and Treatment.* When the hot flashes are eliminated, sleep problems are less common.

• **Formication.** This, the sensation of something crawling on your skin, and itching and dizziness are three other vasomotor effects.

Genitourinary Symptoms

Genitourinary symptoms usually develop later than vasomotor symptoms. Rather than occurring in response to plummeting estrogen levels, genitourinary symptoms develop after estrogen levels have remained low for months or years. Genitourinary symptoms are a reflection of the atrophic (degenerative) changes in the body that occur once a woman's ovaries stop making estradiol. (We discussed the shrinking of reproductive organs in Chapter 1.) Genitourinary symptoms include:

• **Dryness, itching and a sensation of burning in the vagina.** These result from low levels of estrogen in the body. When estradiol levels decline, the cervix (the bottom of the uterus that extends into the vagina) slows down its production of cervical mucus, making the vagina drier. The vaginal wall also thins. When this happens, bumping or rubbing the vagina walls, whether by douching or during sexual intercourse, may cause light bleeding. Vaginal dryness can make sex unpleasant or painful.

• **More frequent urination.** This results when the tissues lining the urethra shrink and become brittle after estrogen levels fall. Some women experience **nocturia** (excessive urination at night). Occasionally urination may be painful.

• **Vaginal infections (vaginitis) and urinary tract infections.** These infections often become more frequent after menopause. The vagina's pH (acid balance) changes after menopause, becoming less acidic and thus making the vagina more hospitable to bacteria that cause vaginal infections. The thinning and shortening of the urinary tract (two of the atrophic changes caused by low estrogen levels) make it easier for bacteria to reach and flourish in the urethra.

Hormone replacement is offered as a way to combat genitourinary symptoms. According to an article in the June 1993 *NARD Journal,* vaginal **atrophy** reverses after approximately one month of HRT, leading to fewer episodes of vaginitis and painful intercourse.

Hormone replacement's effects on urinary symptoms are less clear. Most doctors claim that it works, based on experience with patients (known in medical lingo as "clinical experience"). An analysis of 23 studies evaluating the effectiveness of HRT in treating urinary incontinence, published in *Obstetrics & Gynecology* (January 1994), found only "subjective" improvements. The data "seem to support the impression of benefit of estrogen therapy" for urinary incontinence, the authors of the analysis write, and "no evidence was shown to contradict its use." The American College of Obstetricians and Gynecologists 1992 Technical Bulletin on HRT reports that only one randomized clinical trial demonstrates estrogen's effectiveness in handling urinary tract symptoms—although the bulletin asserts that it is "likely that properly designed studies will confirm a beneficial reduction in the symptoms of urgency, nocturia and frequency in some postmenopausal women with estrogen replacement."

Doctors generally prescribe the pill or patch form of

HRT to alleviate vasomotor and genitourinary discomforts. The estrogens in pills and patches have **systemic** effects—meaning the estrogen circulates via the bloodstream to many areas of the body. But genitourinary problems can persist even when a woman takes estrogen pills or patches. In such cases a practitioner may prescribe a vaginal estrogen cream, which has a **local** effect: It delivers the estrogen directly to organs in the pelvic region. Estrogen creams have a much smaller systemic effect.

Other Symptoms

Other symptoms linked to menopause are neither vasomotor nor genitourinary symptoms. Hormone replacement therapy is sometimes promoted as a medication to treat these problems—although it is debatable whether they are really problems per se. For instance:

• **Thin, less elastic skin.** When estrogen levels decline, skin becomes thinner and loses some elasticity as well as some **collagen** content. (Collagen acts like a padding under the skin, making the skin more resilient.)

Estrogen replacement has been shown in studies to increase the thickness and collagen content of the skin. Some doctors extrapolate from this and say that estrogen will keep the skin looking youthful: "Systemic estrogen use can retard the wrinkling and thinning of the skin that occurs postmenopausally," writes Daniel R. Mishell, Jr., M.D., in *Conn's Current Therapy 1995.*

However, no studies prove that estrogen use (and the resulting thicker collagen content and increased moisture retention) will undo the influence of other factors that age skin and reduce its elasticity—factors such as heredity, cigarette smoking, sun exposure, climate and overall health.

• **Mood changes and depression.** Irritability, anxiety, depression and inability to concentrate have all been blamed on the menopausal years. How much of this is due to a lack of estrogen and how much to other stresses in a woman's life is a matter of lively debate.

Contrary to a centuries-old belief, says health reporter Jane Brody, writing in the September 21, 1994, *New York Times,* numerous studies have determined that "in otherwise emotionally healthy women, menopause by itself does not cause depression." Negative emotional feelings at menopause, Brody's sources suggest, result from having to cope with distressing symptoms such as hot flushes, night sweats, vaginal dryness—things that make you feel you have lost control of your body—as well as from fears of old age or other stresses that contribute to depression. No study proves that lack of estrogen causes mood changes.

Nonetheless, Brody notes, you might feel more positive when taking HRT, "not because it cures depression, but because of its effect on the other symptoms of menopause." It is partly for this reason that HRT proponents advocate hormone replacement as a way of improving a woman's state of mind. Remember, though, that you may be able to achieve the same benefits through nonhormonal or non-drug approaches.

The Many Faces and Forms of HRT

Estrogen and progestin come in many shapes and sizes. Here's a description of what's available on the market and what's coming:

Estrogens

• **Oral estrogen.** The most popular form of estrogen is pill or tablet. When swallowed, oral estrogen is absorbed by the stomach and the intestines, which send the estrogen via the bloodstream to the liver, where it is converted into estrone and then distributed to the tissues in the body.

Oral estrogen is the most commonly used form of estrogen because it's easy to use. Women with stomach or intestinal disorders, however, may not be able to absorb enough estrogen to make HRT effective. And because oral estrogen stimulates the liver, estrogen pills may be unsuitable for women with liver disease, gallbladder disease or blood-clotting disorders. These women may choose to use the newer form of estrogen, the patch, or one of the other estrogen products.

• **Transdermal estrogen.** Sold as Estraderm, the transdermal skin patch is applied much like a Band-Aid to the stomach, hip, thigh or back. Changed once or twice a week, the patch slowly releases estrogen, which is absorbed directly into the bloodstream without first passing through the liver.

Because the liver is bypassed, there is no apparent change in clotting factors (naturally occurring chemicals that affect the formation of blood clots) or in liver proteins, according to the *Physicians' Desk Reference,* the medical industry bible of prescription drug uses, side effects and contraindications. For this reason the patch is thought to be a better route for women who previously couldn't take estrogen pills because the pills aggravate medical conditions such as liver disease, high blood pressure, gallbladder disease and **thrombophlebitis** (a blood clot and an inflammation in a vein such as in a leg). The patch can also be used by women who would simply prefer applying a patch to taking a daily pill.

Wearing the patch day in and day out (which is how it must be used) can irritate the skin. You may need to pull off the patch and reapply it to tougher skin on the buttocks or back. Adhesion may be a problem during hot, humid weather; you must reapply or replace the patch if it falls off.

• **Vaginal estrogen cream.** Vaginal estrogen cream is inserted into the vagina by means of an applicator that dispenses a measured amount of cream—much in the same manner that a woman uses a contraceptive cream or jelly.

Like transdermal estrogen, vaginally applied estrogen is not absorbed through the digestive system and so does not pass through the liver, meaning that it is less likely to aggravate such medical conditions as liver disease, gallbladder disease and thrombophlebitis.

Although some of the estrogen in the cream is absorbed into the bloodstream, most of it remains in the area of the vagina and urinary tract, helping to keep the tissues of the vagina and bladder firm and resilient and combating vaginal dryness and urinary tract infections in the years after menopause. Most of the effects of vaginal creams are local—that is, working primarily in the area in which they are applied. For that reason vaginal creams are not effective in relieving menopausal discomforts such as hot flashes or night sweats or in fighting osteoporosis and heart disease.

• **Suppositories.** Vaginal suppositories made of micronized (finely ground) estrogen can be placed in the vagina. They can be used instead of vaginal creams and serve the same functions: to help keep the tissues of the vagina and bladder firm and to combat vaginal dryness and urinary tract infections.

• **Intramuscular estrogen injections.** In the past, women who couldn't take estrogen orally might be given estrogen injections into a muscle. Injections are rarely used today, made archaic by the advent of the transdermal patch.

• **Implanted subcutaneous estrogen pellets.** Estrogen pellets are one of the new ways of delivering estrogen to the bloodstream while bypassing the liver. Used in Europe (where drugs undergo a shorter laboratory testing process than drugs in the United States), the pellets or capsules are surgically implanted just under the skin. They slowly release estrogen for six to 12 months. If you want to go off the hormone, however, the implant must be surgically removed. At the time of the writing of this book, this estrogen-delivery system is undergoing clinical trials and is not approved for use in the United States.

• **Buccal estrogen.** This is a low-dose estrogen tablet that you place inside your mouth, against your cheek. As it dissolves, the estrogen is absorbed through the mucous membranes into the bloodstream. These tablets are pending approval by the Food and Drug Administration for sale in the United States. They are in use in Europe.

• **Estragel.** In France women use an estrogen gel that is measured with an applicator and then rubbed on the abdomen. The estrogen is absorbed through the skin into the bloodstream. Again, this drug is not yet available in the United States.

• **Vaginal ring implant.** This new estrogen product is inserted in the vagina and left there to slowly release estradiol into the vagina. Vaginal rings are not yet available in the United States.

Progesterones

Regardless of the form it comes in, estrogen can encourage the buildup of endometrial tissue, sometimes leading to hyperplasia. If you have a uterus, you'll probably need to take progestin to prevent hyperplasia. There are two ways to do this:

• **Oral progestins.** Hormone replacement therapy, as practiced today, usually entails supplementing estrogen with a progestin taken in pill form. The most commonly prescribed progestin is medroxyprogesterone.

• **Suppositories.** Progestin suppositories are available for women unable to take oral progestin. For instance, some women have stomach or intestinal disorders that prevent them from absorbing enough of the oral medication.

Short-Term Side Effects of HRT

Hormones are powerful drugs, so it should come as no surprise to you that relief of menopausal symptoms comes with a catch—side effects.

Fifty percent of women taking the most common form of HRT, combination hormone therapy (that is, both estrogen and progestin), experience at least one of the following side effects: water retention, bloating, breast tenderness, feelings of irritability, lower abdominal cramps and irregular, menstrual-like bleeding. Women taking estrogen alone experience similar, though often less extensive, side effects.

Some reactions are eliminated by adjusting (usually reducing) the dose of estrogen and/or progestin. Other reactions disappear after six to eight months of hormone use as your body adjusts to the new types of drugs in its system.

Still other side effects can be managed through diet and exercise or by taking additional medications. All of them disappear if you stop taking HRT.

Let's look at hormone replacement's short-term side effects more closely:

• **Withdrawal bleeding.** If you are taking combination therapy in a cyclic or sequential regimen—that is, estrogen with progestin on certain days of the month—then your most prominent side effect will be the return of your menstrual periods. Doctors call this "withdrawal bleeding" because it occurs after progestin is discontinued, or withdrawn, each month. Eighty to 90 percent of women who begin taking cyclic estrogen plus progestin regain their periods.

The bleeding mimics the menstrual period you had when you were younger. Each month withdrawal bleeding removes the buildup of blood and endometrial tissue caused by taking estrogen, thus cleaning your uterus. These periods generally last from two to five days and gradually lighten over time. After six months or a year of HRT, for instance, you may experience only a couple of days of spotting. Eventually the periods disappear.

Does regaining your period mean you can bear children? No—because HRT won't reactivate your ovaries once they have stopped releasing eggs.

As you can imagine, most women are not keen to resume their menstrual periods. Bleeding is listed as the primary reason women decide not to begin HRT as well as the major reason for discontinuing it.

• **Breakthrough bleeding.** For women who take both estrogen and progestin, an increasingly popular HRT regimen is the continuous combined therapy, in which small

(continued on page 71)

▌ Estrogen Alone or With Progestin?

Research has shown that women with a uterus who take unopposed estrogen (estrogen alone) run a higher risk of developing hyperplasia (a proliferation of endometrial cells) and endometrial cancer (a risk we discuss at length in Chapter 5). To protect against hyperplasia and endometrial cancer, practitioners began prescribing progestin in combination with estrogen.

These widely held beliefs about the risks of endometrial cancer posed by unopposed estrogen may not be well founded, says Howard L. Judd, M.D., professor of obstetrics and gynecology at the University of California (Los Angeles) School of Medicine, in the pages of *Obstetrics and Gynecology News* (December 1993). Judd argues that there are potential errors or flaws in the way in which a substantial number of the most frequently cited pro-progestin studies were conducted. Endometrial cancer is being found in women taking combined estrogen and progestin, Judd says, adding that because of this, views toward progestin's role in hormone replacement therapy may change in the next few years.

The major reason for dropping progestin from HRT is progestin's adverse effects. Some women have such severe side effects from the progestin (chronic headaches, nausea, cramps, depression) that stopping progestin becomes a necessity, asserts Judd. He argues that it is safe to use estrogen-only therapy as long as you are followed carefully by your practitioner and you receive regular endometrial biopsies.

The American College of Obstetricians and Gynecologists, in its HRT Technical Bulletin for its physician

▼

members, acknowledges that estrogen-only therapy can be given to women with a uterus, but an endometrial biopsy should be performed before beginning HRT and every year afterwards. If hyperplasia develops, the bulletin says, estrogen therapy must be discontinued or progestin added. A repeat biopsy is needed to be sure the hyperplasia has cleared up.

doses of progestin are taken along with estrogen all month long. In contrast, the three other forms of estrogen-progestin therapy entail taking progestin only on certain days of the month. (See Chapter 1 for a review of these regimens.) When using the continuous combined therapy, you may have light menstrual-like spotting (breakthrough bleeding) during the first six months of treatment. But because you take progestin continually, you won't experience the two or three days of withdrawal bleeding of women on the cyclic combined regimen (*Annals of Internal Medicine,* December 12, 1992).

Report any breakthrough bleeding to your doctor, who may decide to adjust the ratio of estrogen to progestin. If the bleeding lasts more than 10 days or is heavier than your normal menstrual period ever was, your doctor may want to perform tests such as an endometrial biopsy or an ultrasound to rule out cervical polyps (small, usually noncancerous growths), uterine **fibroids** (noncancerous muscle and tissue growths) or hyperplasia (a dangerous buildup of tissue in the uterus that can set the stage for cancer). Abnormal bleeding—that is, any unscheduled bleeding—is not a good thing.

• **Water retention and bloating.** Half of the women who take HRT experience fluid retention or a feeling of gas and bloatedness, caused by both estrogen and progestin. If these side effects don't pass in a few weeks, and you find them bothersome, speak to your doctor. She may adjust your hormone dose, suggest reducing your intake of salt and caffeine (which encourage water retention), offer a prescription **diuretic** (a drug that promotes the production and discharge of urine) or recommend taking a small amount of a natural diuretic, such as vitamin B_6.

• **Breast swelling and tenderness.** Women who take HRT often develop swollen and tender breasts, similar to premenstrual breast tenderness. Called **mastalgia** in medical lingo, it is thought to be provoked by estrogen and may disappear in a few months. Your doctor might choose to address breast tenderness by lowering your estrogen dose or by prescribing Estratest—a combination of estrogen with testosterone (a male hormone also found in the female body) to relieve painful breasts.

• **Nausea and/or abdominal cramps.** If you're taking progestin with estrogen, you could experience nausea or cramping in the lower abdomen during or after the days you take progestin. Taking smaller progestin doses may eliminate this.

• **Weight gain.** At least 25 percent of women on HRT put on weight, particularly in the breasts, lower abdomen and hips. Some of the gain may be caused by the fluid retained during the first few months using HRT. (Other causes of weight gain are not necessarily attributable to HRT, including a slowdown in the body's metabolism that accompanies aging and a reduction in calorie burning due

(continued on page 74)

▌Testosterone and Its Effects on the Female Body

Testosterone, a male hormone or androgen, is prescribed to menopausal or postmenopausal women for two reasons: It counters persistent, uncomfortable side effects of estrogen, particularly breast tenderness; and it increases libido, or sexual desire.

Testosterone has a few side effects of its own: cosmetic side effects and **lipid** (blood fats) side effects:

Cosmetic effects include voice deepening and facial **hirsutism** (excessive hair growth on the upper lip or chin). These effects occur in 15 to 20 percent of women who receive high doses of male hormones (150 mg of injectable testosterone monthly), according to Gloria A. Bachmann, M.D., professor of obstetrics and gynecology at the University of Medicine and Dentistry of New Jersey, writing in *The Female Patient* (July 1993). When the testosterone dose was cut in half (75 mg a month), hirsutism occurred in less than 5 percent of the women.

Testosterone doses given in HRT, taken orally every day, are designed to be low dose (1.25 or 2.5 mg a day) and to give relief to menopausal symptoms in about three weeks. Cosmetic side effects are rare, says Ronald L. Young, M.D., associate professor of obstetrics and gynecology at Baylor College of Medicine in Houston. Reducing the dose of testosterone will usually quickly reverse the cosmetic side effects.

Lipid effects of testosterone are possible in the form of a change in cholesterol levels. Testosterone, when taken at high doses, appears to lower HDL ("good") cholesterol levels. Although lower HDL levels are most

▼

common when androgens are taken in high doses, the decrease in HDL cholesterol has also been reported in women on low doses of testosterone. Whether or not the testosterone-caused cholesterol changes translate to an increase in heart disease is not yet known. (We address cholesterol and issues of HRT and heart disease in Chapter 4.)

to a lower level of exercise.) Some doctors believe that estrogen itself tends to encourage the development of fat tissue. Adjusting hormone doses may or may not help.

• **Chronic headaches.** Women on HRT report that they develop chronic headaches. Researchers think that the cause is fluid retention in the brain. Usually the headaches disappear after three or four months of therapy. If they continue, however, your doctor may need to reduce the amount of estrogen you're taking.

If you are prone to migraine headaches, the estrogen in HRT may increase the number of migraines you experience. If so, it may be necessary to take you off estrogen altogether. (See the discussion of migraines and hormone replacement therapy in this chapter.)

• **Depression and irritability.** These are just the kinds of emotional upheavals that some advocates claim HRT will solve! If you find yourself depressed or irritated after beginning HRT, your doctor may choose to reduce your progestin dose, have you try a different form of progestin or give you a prescription for natural progesterone (which must be prepared by a pharmacist). Natural progesterone is thought to be less likely to provoke depression than synthetic progestin.

In fact, trying different forms of estrogen and progestin may be useful in addressing all HRT side effects. Writing in the December 15, 1992, *Annals of Internal Medicine,* Deborah Grady, M.D., and her colleagues on the American College of Physicians Clinical Efficacy Assessment Subcommittee report that side effects as varied as depression, irritability, bloating and breast tenderness are less often a problem in women taking low-dose daily progestins and

▌HRT and Men

Your use of hormone replacement therapy can affect the health of your male partner if you're using estrogen cream shortly before intercourse.

Morris Notelovitz, M.D., read a report in the medical literature of breast enlargement in a man whose wife used estrogen cream as a vaginal lubricant before sex. To gauge the short-term side effects of estrogen creams on a woman's husband or partner, Notelovitz conducted a small study of men and estrogen creams. Describing his study in his book *Menopause and Midlife Health,* Notelovitz found that blood levels of estrogen doubled in men and blood levels of androgen (male hormone) fell 50 percent in men two hours after the men applied estrogen creams to their penises. All levels returned to normal after 24 hours.

There's no evidence that male breast enlargement is a widespread problem among the partners of women using vaginal estrogen creams. Nonetheless, Notelovitz suggests that you not use estrogen creams as a vaginal lubricant for intercourse.

in women taking natural progesterone.

Other reported reactions to HRT include nausea, rashes, increased appetite, increased vaginal secretions, lowered levels of sexual desire and—conversely—heightened sexual desire. Clearly there's a great and even conflicting range of side effects that you may experience. The point is, watch for them and ask your doctor to take action if you suspect a problem.

Who Cannot Take HRT? Absolute and Not-So-Absolute Contraindications

If you have menopausal symptoms, does that mean you need HRT? Some doctors will say yes. Only you, however, can decide how annoying or disruptive the problems are, whether you want to address them with a pharmaceutical approach like HRT, use other methods to manage the symptoms or simply wait them out.

If you try HRT and don't like the side effects, there's nothing to say that you have to continue taking it. Discuss the situation with your doctor, who can propose alternatives and recommend ways to gently phase off of HRT. Don't, however, adjust your medication without your doctor's approval—that can be dangerous. If you still have your uterus, for example, it's risky to stop taking your progestin and take unopposed estrogen. Even if you dislike the side effects of the progestin portion of HRT, estrogen taken alone is not a good idea unless you have an annual endometrial biopsy or similar test to ensure your endometrium remains healthy.

That said, there are times when practitioners will strongly recommend HRT. Usually these times involve situations of premature menopause, in which a woman in her

20s or 30s has lost her ovaries through surgery or her ovaries have become damaged and have stopped producing estrogen. Current medical wisdom says that a woman who loses the protective benefits of her estrogen at such an early age is at risk of developing osteoporosis or heart disease as early as in her 50s.

Are there times when a woman absolutely should not take HRT? Yes. HRT is inappropriate if you have certain medical conditions. In medical parlance these conditions are known as **absolute contraindications** to HRT.

Over time, the number of absolute contraindications has been whittled down. There were approximately 15 absolute contraindications 20 years ago; today there are fewer absolute contraindications and relative contraindications.

The primary reason for so many changes from absolute to relative is that estrogen doses in HRT have been getting smaller, and most estrogens used in HRT today are natural estrogens rather than synthetic. Medical researchers believe these low-dose natural estrogens are safer than the estrogens of 30 years ago.

Another big change in HRT options arrived when the transdermal skin patch came on the market. The transdermal patch delivers estrogen directly into the bloodstream, bypassing the digestive system and the liver, making it less apt to aggravate such medical conditions as liver dysfunction, gallbladder disease and blood-clotting problems. Many doctors consider the patch safer than taking estrogen orally for women with certain health problems.

So what absolute contraindications still exist? According to the American College of Obstetricians and Gynecologists 1992 Technical Bulletin on hormone replacement therapy,

(continued on page 79)

▋ Your Personal Risks

To help you keep track of your personal risks, we've prepared this checklist. As you read this chapter, tick off those conditions or situations that apply to you. Use this checklist as a jumping-off point for discussions about hormone replacement therapy between you and your health care practitioner.

Conditions that ABSOLUTELY contraindicate HRT

- ☐ Personal or family history of breast cancer
- ☐ Personal history of endometrial cancer
- ☐ History of thrombosis (blood clotting), including heart attacks or strokes caused by blood clots
- ☐ Active liver disease
- ☐ Impaired liver function
- ☐ Unexplained vaginal bleeding

Conditions that MAY contraindicate HRT

- ☐ High blood pressure
- ☐ Gallbladder disease
- ☐ Diabetes mellitus
- ☐ Fibroids
- ☐ Migraines
- ☐ Endometriosis
- ☐ Seizure disorders
- ☐ Congestive heart failure
- ☐ Family history of very high blood cholesterol
- ☐ DES use by you or your mother

women with breast cancer, endometrial cancer, a recent history of blood clots, liver disease or impaired liver function and unexplained vaginal bleeding should not take HRT. If any of these apply to you and your doctor suggests HRT, be sure you sit down for a serious discussion. These are issues you should cover in your powwow.

Absolute Contraindications

There are several conditions that flash a red light to any women considering HRT:

History of certain cancers. HRT is off-limits for women with breast cancer or with endometrial cancer (uterine cancer), says the American College of Obstetricians and Gynecologists. The *Cecil Textbook of Medicine* cites malignant melanoma (a form of skin cancer) as another absolute contraindication, and other sources add kidney tumors to this list. Tumors of the breast, uterus or kidney can be estrogen dependent—meaning that they grow when they are fed by estrogen. In these cases HRT must be avoided. If you were successfully treated for estrogen-dependent breast cancer 10, 15, 20 years before your menopause, it's prudent to avoid HRT. There is very little evidence showing that women taking HRT have a recurrence of breast cancer, but few women and their medical practitioners want to take the risk.

Some cancers are not estrogen dependent. In such cases some doctors are willing to offer a woman a short course of HRT (one or two years) if hot flashes and other menopausal discomforts are unbearable. The general consensus, however, is that women with previous cancer should not take hormone therapy.

What if you are at high risk for breast cancer or endometrial cancer? Should you go on HRT in the first place?

A strong family history of breast cancer is an absolute contra-indication to HRT, says Isaac Schiff, M.D., chief of gynecology service at Massachusetts General Hospital, in *Modern Medicine* (January 1993). A family history of endometrial cancer is not considered an absolute contraindication.

Recent history of deep-vein blood clots. A recent history of **thrombosis** (abnormal, deep-vein clotting) is an absolute contraindication to HRT. Estrogen has been shown to decrease the anticlotting factors of the blood, so that women on HRT who tend to develop clots might experience thrombophlebitis (a blood clot and an inflammation in a vein such as in a leg) or **thromboembolism** (a clot that breaks away and travels to the lungs, heart or brain, where it blocks a blood vessel). This situation could lead to heart attack or stroke, among other dangerous conditions.

Varicose veins and hemorrhoids are not considered contraindications to HRT. Although these conditions are caused by blood clots, the clots are in the veins on the surface of the body, not in the deep veins. Varicose veins and hemorrhoids don't pose the same risk of stroke or heart attack as thromboembolism.

What if you had thrombophlebitis in the past, but have had no problems in recent years—could you use HRT? Not if hormone use triggered the condition in the past. If previous thrombophlebitis was not hormone related, the answer is less clear. The American College of Obstetricians and Gynecologists Technical Bulletin warns physicians that "the risk posed by estrogen use in a patient with a past episode of thrombosis is unknown." A conservative physician may well consider estrogen use too risky for a woman with a history of deep-vein clotting. Other practitioners believe that the new transdermal patch or a vaginal estrogen cream are two options for women susceptible to clotting, as long as those women are given blood tests to be sure their anti-clotting factors are normal. Research published in the December 1993 *American Journal of Obstetrics and Gynecology* confirmed the hypothesis that current doses of HRT do not appear to cause blood clots.

Active liver disease or impaired liver function. When estrogen is taken orally, it is processed by the liver before it goes into the bloodstream. An impaired or diseased liver may not convert estrogen properly; in turn, the estrogen may become a toxin in the body. The American College of Obstetricians and Gynecologists lists active liver disease and chronic (long-lasting) impaired liver function as contraindications to estrogen replacement therapy.

A past history of liver disease is not an absolute contraindication for HRT. Some doctors believe that vaginal estrogen creams and transdermal patches are safe for women who do not have active liver disease, because the estrogen in the creams and patches are *not* taken orally and thus the estrogen bypasses the liver.

Undiagnosed vaginal bleeding. If you are bleeding and don't know why, you shouldn't start HRT before your doctor investigates and addresses the problem. Vaginal bleeding can signal uterine fibroids (noncancerous growths in uterine muscle tissue), hyperplasia (a proliferation of cells inside the uterus), uterine cancer or cervical cancer. Estrogen can make these conditions worse. Undiagnosed bleeding may be eliminated as a contraindication if your practitioner identifies the cause and finds that it is not affected by hormone use.

Relative Contraindications

Beyond the absolute contraindications are situations in which HRT use must be weighed carefully. Some doctors call these **relative contraindications**. Estrogen sometimes—but not always—worsens these medical conditions.

If you have one of the following conditions, and you elect to take hormones, proceed with care. Work with your doctor to weigh the severity of your menopausal symptoms and the therapy's potential benefits in light of the following known risks. And make sure your doctor closely monitors your use of hormones and is ready to modify your regimen if problems arise.

• **High blood pressure.** Estrogen encourages the kidneys to produce **angiotensin**, a chemical that causes blood vessels to narrow. In turn, blood pressure can increase, a situation that doctors call "estrogen-associated hypertension."

Estrogen-associated high blood pressure is a problem caused by oral contraceptives, but the evidence is less clear for HRT. Of several studies published between 1976 and 1988, says the American College of Obstetricians and Gynecologists 1992 Technical Bulletin, only two studies were able to link hormone replacement with increased blood pressure, and that link was in women whose blood pressure was already high before therapy began.

If you are already hypertensive, no one can say how your body will react to HRT. Again this is something for you and your doctor to monitor.

• **Gallbladder disease.** Estrogen, particularly oral estrogen, has been linked to increased incidence of gallbladder disease, according to *Current Obstetric and Gynecologic Diagnosis and Treatment*. Estrogen causes increased amounts of cholesterol to collect in the **bile** manufactured by the liver. The bile becomes supersaturated with cholesterol, and gallstones (three-quarters of which are composed primarily of cholesterol) form.

Thus, estrogen in the form of pills and tablets is usually off-limits to women with gallbladder problems. Transdermal patches and vaginal creams are thought to be safe options because, as we've mentioned already, the estrogen is absorbed into the bloodstream through the skin and doesn't pass through the liver. If you have a history of gallbladder disease or gallstones and you choose to try HRT, be sure your doctor monitors the effects of therapy on your body through blood tests. An ultrasound test or a special x-ray called a cholecystogram can make a diagnosis if gallstones are suspected.

• **Diabetes mellitus.** If you have an undiagnosed case of diabetes, HRT may be the trigger that brings it to your attention, says Lois Jovanovic, M.D., in *Hormones: The Woman's Answerbook*. She advises that if diabetes develops during hormone replacement, the therapy should be stopped.

Estrogen, even in the low doses found in hormone replacement, can disturb blood sugar levels. Jovanovic states that a woman with previously diagnosed diabetes can take HRT as long as she increases her dose of insulin and she doesn't have any of the severe complications of diabetes such as eye, kidney or foot problems.

• **Fibroids.** Fibroids are benign (noncancerous) tumors found in or on the uterus. Twenty percent of all women have fibroids, as do half of women over age 50. Fibroids usually shrink on their own after menopause, when estrogen levels fall, says Sadja Greenwood, M.D., author of

Menopause Naturally, Updated: Preparing for the Second Half of Life.

Fibroids are seldom troublesome. You might have one or more (they occur in clusters) and not even know it because you feel no symptoms or ill effect. Sometimes, though, fibroids cause heavy bleeding during your menstrual cycle, cause pain or put uncomfortable pressure on your bladder or bowel. If fibroids grow large enough (three and one-half inches or more in diameter) or cause you pain, doctors may recommend surgery to remove the fibroids or an estrogen-blocking drug to shrink them.

Because estrogen stimulates fibroid growth, some women with large fibroids choose not to take HRT. Other women with fibroids wait two or three years before starting HRT to give their fibroids time to wither and shrink. Still other women are willing to try low-dose hormone replacement, particularly if their fibroids are small and not troublesome. If while on HRT you develop fibroids that cause heavy bleeding, abdominal pain or uncomfortable pressure on your bladder or bowel, then you'll have to discontinue HRT. You probably won't be able to resume estrogen use.

• **Migraine headaches.** Estrogen replacement in menopause can provoke migraine headaches. Reducing the amount of estrogen you take may solve the problem. But if your migraines persist several weeks after trying a lowered dose, you may decide the benefits of hormone use are not worth the pain in the form of migraines.

New research note: Some of the latest research claims that a tendency to migraine headaches is one of the uncontrollable risks for stroke, along with such uncontrollable risks as age, sex, race and family history of stroke. Do migraines cause stroke? No. They are simply an indication of a possible increase in stroke risk. However, be aware that the link between migraines, HRT and stroke has not been studied.

• **Endometriosis.** This occurs when cells from the endometrium (the tissue lining the uterus) migrate outside the uterus, where they grow on other organs within the abdomen when stimulated by the menstrual cycle.

Endometriosis can be quite painful. Before menopause, treatment for this condition involves taking doses of estrogen, progestin and sometimes other hormones. If these don't work, the uterus, fallopian tubes and ovaries may be surgically removed. After menopause, less severe endometriosis may disappear when estrogen and progesterone levels fall. For that reason doctors often withhold HRT from women with endometriosis for three to 12 months after menopause. The idea is to give the migrated endometrial cells time to wither and die so that the woman can then use estrogen without stimulating the migrated cells.

Other conditions considered to be relative contraindications include seizure disorders, congestive heart failure, a family history of very high blood cholesterol levels, and a history of diethylstilbestrol (DES, a potent estrogen) used by you or your mother.

The medical profession has been gradually enlarging its definition of women who are candidates for HRT and shrinking the list of women who "absolutely cannot" take HRT. Be aware that in medical parlance "absolute" is not always as hard and fast as you would think. In the words of the *Cecil Textbook of Medicine,* "Individual exceptions to even the absolute contraindications exist." What this means it that you have a doubly confusing but crucial job as a medical consumer—making sure your health care practitioner clarifies the reasons why you can (or cannot) take HRT.

Approach your evaluation of HRT as an informed consumer. Do any absolute or relative contraindications apply to you? Would you feel comfortable taking HRT under one of these situations? Would you feel more comfortable seeking other methods of treatment?

Your answers will depend on many factors: how debilitating your menopausal symptoms are; whether you plan to take HRT for short-term treatment of symptoms or to arrest long-term bone loss (see Chapter 4); what your doctor suggests; and even how comfortable you are following a medication schedule and participating in the extra monitoring that HRT under these conditions warrants.

How Much Estrogen Should You Take?

In general the medical philosophy is that you should take the lowest dose that works. The more estrogen and progestin you take, the greater your risks of developing uncomfortable and potentially dangerous side effects. The American College of Obstetricians and Gynecologists recommends that doctors start women at the low-dose standard of .625 mg once a day of conjugated estrogen or its equivalent in other forms. This dose, the college writes in its 1992 Technical Bulletin, is effective in alleviating many of the symptoms of menopause. It also happens to be the lowest dose shown to prevent osteoporosis. This is good if bone loss is a concern for you. (You get a chance to evaluate this concern in Chapter 4.) If osteoporosis is not an issue, you may be able to take a smaller amount of estrogen. Some women find relief of menopausal symptoms with only .3 mg of estrogen a day.

You may surmise that the standard dose has been arrived at through extensive scientific research. That's only partly true. Yes, the studies have shown that .625 mg of conjugated estrogen is the lowest level for arresting bone loss. But no studies have proven that this dose is *best* for short-term HRT use. As Lynn Rosenberg, Sc.D., writes in the December 1993 *American Journal of Public Health,* "There are many unanswered questions about how long estrogens must be taken to achieve a beneficial effect, how soon an effect dissipates after discontinuation, what doses of estrogen are effective and which groups of women benefit."

Do all women take the standard .625 mg dose? No. The most commonly prescribed form of oral estrogen is conjugated estrogen (sold as Premarin), which is offered in a so-called very low dose .3 mg, the standard dose .625 mg, and in two larger doses: .9 mg and 1.25 mg. Women with severe hot flashes may require high doses—2.25 mg or 5 mg—for a short time, although the American College of Obstetricians and Gynecologists recommends that these high doses be gradually reduced to the standard dose.

There are several factors that influence what is the right dose for you:

How much estrogen your body produced during the reproductive years. If your practitioner knows how much estrogen previously circulated through your bloodstream, then it will be easier to determine what level of estrogen therapy to try. The only way to know this number is if your blood is tested for estradiol levels before you enter the menopausal years. If you've already started experiencing menopause, it's too late to make those measurements.

Your age. Younger women may need twice as much estrogen as older women to alleviate symptoms, says the

Cecil Textbook of Medicine.

Your weight. Heavier women may need a smaller dose because they have more estrone, the estrogen produced from fat cells, in their bodies than thinner women.

Whether your menopause was surgical or natural. Women who have had their ovaries surgically removed may need higher estrogen amounts. Because of the suddenness of surgical menopause, these women tend to have more severe menopausal symptoms than women who have had natural menopause.

Whether you smoke. Smoking has been found to reduce the amounts of estradiol and estrone in the blood, so cigarette smokers on HRT appear to need a higher dose of estrogen, according to research published in *Obstetrics and Gynecology* (June 1993).

Your body's sensitivity to estrogen in general. You can only determine this by trying the standard dose of estrogen and seeing how you react. If you are still experiencing side effects such as headache or breast pain or swelling after four months, you may need a lower dose or a different estrogen formulation. Each pharmaceutical estrogen— micronized, conjugated, esterified, transdermal—has a different formulation and affects women slightly differently. (See Chapter 1 for a review of estrogens on the market.) If you take HRT and it doesn't relieve your symptoms, your doctor may up the dosage for several months.

Finding the precise dose of estrogen (and the ratio of progestin to estrogen, if you take a combined therapy) that works for you is part science and part guesswork. The medical establishment calls it an "empiric" process—meaning trial and error in the consumer's vocabulary.

The Progestin Connection

How much progestin should you take? If you are on the cyclic sequential regimen, the rule of thumb is 5 to 10 mg of a progestin such as medroxyprogesterone acetate (now the progestin of choice, according to the American College of Obstetricians and Gynecologists) taken for 10 or 14 consecutive days of the month. If you are on the continuous combined regimen, you may be prescribed 10 mg, 5 mg or 2.5 mg a day throughout the month. The 10 mg dose is thought to provide the best protection against developing hyperplasia and endometrial cancer, but it also causes more side effects—such as the headaches and depression that we discussed earlier. Reaching the right balance of estrogen and progestin may require some dose adjustments in the first few months of treatment.

How Long Should You Take HRT?

If you are taking hormones strictly to alleviate menopausal symptoms (and not as possible protection against heart disease and osteoporosis), then HRT should be given for a limited time—as brief as one but no more than five years, according to the American College of Physicians guidelines published in the December 15, 1992, *Annals of Internal Medicine.* Toward the end of this period, your practitioner may gradually reduce your dose of estrogen. An abrupt halt—with a corresponding plunge in estrogen levels—could make menopausal symptoms recur. Even with a tapered dose, though, some women experience such symptoms again once they have stopped therapy. (In Chapter 5 we cover the who, what, when, why and how of stopping HRT.)

If all you want is assistance through your first meno-pausal years, a helping hand to soothe hot flashes and let you gradually phase into your postmenopausal years, short-term HRT may be a boon. If you want to take hormones for their possible protection against osteoporosis and heart disease, then your doctor will recommend taking hormones for longer than five years. Whichever path you choose (and you can always change your mind), you'll want to develop a good partnership with the person who provides your health care.

Who Provides HRT

In your hunt for more information on hormone replace-ment therapy, it pays to be working with a medical practi-tioner conversant in the nuances of HRT. But who should that person be? A doctor who specializes in HRT? A family doctor who knows your entire family medical history? A knowledgeable nurse practitioner at a nearby women's health care clinic?

Hormone replacement regimens can be complex. Not only does the practitioner need to select the appropriate form of HRT—pill, patch or cream—for your needs, she also needs to determine the correct dose, monitor any risk factors such as diabetes or cancer and ensure that you are receiving the necessary nutrients (such as calcium) to make HRT effective. In addition, estrogen and progestin doses may change over time. What you receive when you are just beginning menopause, and perhaps coping with hot flashes and night sweats, may be different from what you might take five or 10 years after menopause. These are all good reasons to make sure you're seeing a doctor who knows what she is doing. Here are some of your choices:

• **Obstetrician-gynecologist.** This is an M.D. (doctor of medicine) or D.O. (doctor of osteopathy) trained in all aspects of pregnancy and childbirth (obstetrics) as well as the health and proper functioning of the female reproductive system (gynecology). An obstetrician-gynecologist completes approximately four years of ob-gyn residency training after medical school.

You might choose an ob-gyn for your birth practitioner; select an ob-gyn for routine gynecological care; visit this specialist if you have a specific gynecological problem; or use an ob-gyn as your primary physician, one who treats you for ailments such as the common cold or conditions like diabetes or high blood pressure. Some ob-gyns subspecialize in gynecologic oncology (gynecologic cancers), maternal and fetal medicine (complications of pregnancy) and reproductive endocrinology (hormonal and infertility problems). The latter subspecialty is the most directly related to the issue of hormone replacement.

Obstetrician-gynecologists are more likely to prescribe hormone replacement therapy than any other medical practitioner. Fifty-six to 94 percent of ob-gyns report that they *routinely* prescribe HRT for their postmenopausal patients, according to an analysis of physician surveys published in the *Journal of Women's Health*. (See "Who Prescribes What?" on page 95 for more on physician prescribing habits.) As is true for any health care practitioner you select, find out if your ob-gyn stays up-to-date on the latest HRT research, and be sure the practice includes a large number of women in approximately the same stage of life as you (whether that be perimenopause, menopause itself or **postmenopause**). A doctor whose practice consists mostly of obstetric services, or who primarily treats younger women, may not know enough about the problems of menopause to serve you well.

• **Family practitioner.** You may select a family practitioner for your obstetrical and gynecological care. Family practice is a relatively new medical specialty concerned with the total health care of the individual (woman or man, adult or child) and the family. A family practitioner who is board-certified has three years of training following medical school, including a minimum of one month of gynecology and two months of obstetrics. If you choose a family practitioner to oversee your HRT, be sure the doctor has the knowledge and expertise in gynecology and in health concerns of older women.

• **Internist.** This M.D. or D.O. specializes in the diagnosis and nonsurgical treatment of disease, especially diseases in adults. Many internists set up practices in which they act as highly trained family doctors. However, they often specialize in other areas such as gastroenterology, which deals with disorders of the digestive tract. Internists can provide some routine gynecological care, but be aware that they are not required to have any training in gynecology, although they can elect to take three months of training in ob-gyn during their residency. They may or may not have adequate knowledge of HRT.

• **Endocrinologist.** This doctor is an M.D. or D.O. specially trained in the treatment of hormonal disorders, including problems related to menopause, as well as diabetes, pituitary diseases and sexual problems. The usual track is for the physician to specialize in internal medicine with a subspecialty in endocrinology.

Endocrinologists are not primary care physicians. They

rarely provide routine gynecological or family care, concentrating instead on hormone dysfunctions. Chances are good that if you go to an endocrinologist, it will be at the suggestion of your primary care physician. Be sure your health care practitioner refers you to an endocrinologist who has interest in and experience with treating menopause-related concerns.

• **Homeopathic practitioners.** A **homeopathic physician** treats illnesses by using natural medicines that stimulate a person's own healing powers while avoiding harmful side effects. An M.D. or D.O. can become a homeopathic physician by getting additional training in homeopathic principles. There are over 500 M.D.'s and D.O.'s nationwide who include homeopathic principles in their practice of medicine, according to the National Center for Homeopathy. Other health care practitioners, such as nurse practitioners, nurse-midwives, physician assistants, licensed acupuncturists and **naturopathic** physicians (licensed in eight states to diagnose and treat illness), may be allowed to use homeopathy within the scope of their licenses, depending on the laws of the state in which they reside.

The homeopathic approach to menopause focuses on improving nutrition, exercise and overall health and on correcting any imbalances in the body. Some homeopathic physicians—including Andrew Lockie, M.D., and Nicola Geddes, M.D., authors of *The Women's Guide to Homeopathy*—prescribe HRT for menopausal women, particularly those who have had a surgical menopause. At the same time, Lockie and Geddes are careful not to encourage a woman to use hormone therapy "as a substitute for adopting a healthy lifestyle," they write. A basic tenet of homeopathy is that the whole person must be treated and not just the disease.

• **Nurse practitioner.** As a registered nurse with additional graduate training, a nurse practitioner can give you information about HRT's pros and cons and about health-promoting steps for your postmenopausal years. Licensing laws vary from state to state, but in general you can find a nurse practitioner in an ob-gyn office or at a women's health clinic, performing entire routine gynecological exams, ordering and interpreting routine lab tests, managing minor gynecological problems, providing care for uncomplicated pregnancies as well as prescribing and educating women about following a hormone replacement regimen. Look for a nurse practitioner who has training and experience in gynecological care and who spends enough time with you to answer all your questions.

• **Certified nurse-midwife.** This is a registered nurse who has completed graduate training in women's health, obstetrical care and gynecological care and has passed an extensive credentialing examination administered by the American College of Nurse-Midwives. All 50 states allow certified nurse-midwives to collaborate with physicians, and in 32 states (this number has been increasing every year) certified nurse-midwives have the authority to prescribe oral contraceptives and hormone replacement therapy.

Nurse-midwives practice in a variety of settings: hospitals, birthing centers, health maintenance organizations, public health departments and public and private health clinics. Although midwives in decades (and centuries) past focused on maternity care, today's certified nurse-midwives serve as primary care practitioners, offering a range of gynecological services to women of all ages.

(continued on page 96)

▌ Who Prescribes What?

What are the trends in hormone replacement as prescribed by doctors? An article in the fall 1993 issue of the *Journal of Women's Health* examined this question. Erin K. Scalley, B.S., and Janet B. Henrich, M.D., of the Yale University School of Medicine, reviewed 31 physician surveys published since 1987 to determine prescribing practices. Here are some of the facts they unearthed:

• Fifty-six to 94 percent of gynecologists reported that they *routinely* prescribed hormone replacement therapy to postmenopausal women.

• Fifty to 98 percent of general practitioners and internists reported that they prescribed HRT, though not on a routine basis.

• Women physicians and younger practitioners were more likely to prescribe HRT than male or older practitioners.

• Most gynecologists and general practitioners prescribed estrogen with progestin for women who had a natural menopause.

• Physicians who were older and high prescribers of HRT tended to prescribe estrogen alone to women with a uterus.

• Eighty percent of physicians prescribed an oral estrogen, followed in prescription frequency by the transdermal patch, vaginal estrogen creams and (rarely) injections. Medroxyprogesterone acetate was the most popular progestin prescribed.

Whomever you choose to help you in deciding to take HRT, be sure you ask the practitioner at least the following questions:

- What is your training in women's health?
- How many patients do you have on HRT?
- Why are they on HRT?
- How long do they stay on it?
- What kinds of problems do you see among them?
- Should I be seeing another doctor who specializes in this area?
- What are my risks of developing heart disease or osteoporosis? In light of my personal medical history, will HRT lower those risks?
- What are my risks of developing breast cancer, migraines, gallstones or other health conditions that have been linked to HRT? In light of my personal medical history, will HRT increase those risks?
- Will HRT change my life expectancy? By how much?
- Will you prescribe estrogen with progestin? Why or why not?
- What are the common side effects of the regimen you are recommending?
- Will I experience any bleeding when on HRT and, if so, what should it be like?
- If I take estrogen without progestin, how frequently should I be monitored for hyperplasia and other possible problems? What form will this monitoring take?
- If I decide to try HRT, when should I start?
- How much time do I have to make this decision?

Feel free to add more questions to the list, particularly as they pertain to the long-term benefits and risks of hormone replacement, the subject of the next chapter.

▮ What to Expect in the Doctor's Office

Before you begin hormone replacement, your health care practitioner should conduct a thorough evaluation of your medical history and your current physical condition. This exam shouldn't be a one-time event. A couple of months after beginning HRT, your practitioner will want to touch base with you and probably fine-tune your hormone doses.

The fact is you should be closely monitored by your health care practitioner *for as long as you take HRT.* This means office visits at least once a year; your practitioner may want you to come every six months. Your visits should include:

• A full physical examination, including a pelvic exam and a breast exam

• A Pap smear (also called a cervical smear). This sampling of cervical cells will be shipped to a lab and checked under microscope for signs of cancer and precancerous conditions.

• A blood pressure check

• Blood tests for calcium and phosphorus levels (both important nutrients in preventing bone loss) and cholesterol and triglyceride levels

• If you are on oral estrogen, blood tests for blood sugar, liver function, thyroid function and clotting factors. These monitor any aggravation of health conditions that can be contraindications to HRT.

• A yearly mammogram. This breast x-ray can detect early cancer and is important because of the ongoing controversy about effect of HRT on breast cancer. (Details about this controversy are in Chapter 5.)

▼

• Bone density tests or other tests to measure bone strength if osteoporosis may be a problem

• An endometrial biopsy or an **ultrasound** vaginal probe if you are taking estrogen without progestin and still have a uterus. These measure the health of the endometrium. A precancerous condition can develop in as few as 12 months of unopposed estrogen.

• Possibly an ultrasound examination of the ovaries to look for ovarian cysts and other visible changes in ovarian size or health

In short, as long as you are taking HRT, you will need to be monitored regularly. Some women find that reassuring; other women dislike the bother of office visits and resent what they consider the "medicalization" of a natural process of aging. Yet, in light of the possible negative effects of HRT (which we examine closely in Chapter 5), frequent medical checkups are essential for your well-being and health.

CHAPTER IV

Preventive Hormone Therapy After Menopause

S ome women and their health care practitioners view hormone replacement therapy simply as a treatment for menopausal symptoms such as hot flashes. Increasingly, however, doctors are portraying HRT as a preventive therapy. If it hasn't happened already, you'll probably be asked to consider taking estrogen and its partner, progestin, to help to lower your risk of osteoporosis and heart disease and ward off vaginal and urinary tract infections.

In fact, as soon as you pass through menopause, your doctor may bring up the subject of long-term postmenopausal hormone replacement, particularly if you elect HRT to manage hot flashes and other menopausal symptoms. In the absence of side effects, your doctor may imply that it's an easy matter to simply continue taking your pills or using your creams and patches.

It is in this realm of long-term use of HRT that the greatest debate over hormone use rages. On the one side is the argument that it would be unfair to deprive you of the possible health benefits of a "natural" substance, estrogen, for 20 or 30 years of your life. On the other side is the argument that the safety and need for this drug therapy have not yet been proven and that prescribing drugs to women who are not at risk is not sound medical practice.

In weighing long-term use of hormones—that is, HRT for 10, 20, 30 years or more—you and your doctor need to decide whether you are at risk for the medical conditions that long-term HRT may protect against. Let's look at these conditions now.

Genitourinary Problems

As we saw in Chapter 3, when estrogen levels fall during menopause, the changes affect many parts of the body, including the vagina and the urinary tract.

After menopause, vaginal tissues slowly start to shrink and become dry, thin, less elastic and more susceptible to irritation (a situation called **atrophic vaginitis**). The vagina's pH (acidity balance) rises, becoming more alkaline. The declining acidity level makes the vagina susceptible to inflammation and infection. At the same time, a woman may notice that her body is producing less vaginal lubrication during sex. The medical profession's term for these gradual changes is atrophic changes.

Every woman's reproductive organs begin to atrophy shortly after menopause due to lower estrogen levels. Not every woman experiences problems as a result, however. For those who do, the most common symptom is atrophic vaginitis, and it can continue for life. This distinguishes atrophic vaginitis from transitional menopausal symptoms such as hot flashes, which usually only last a few years as your body adjusts to new, lower levels of estrogen.

For some women an easily irritated vagina combined with little natural lubrication makes sexual intercourse painful. Painful sex may begin five to 10 years after menopause—if it occurs at all.

If you have these problems, you can use nonhormonal lubricating creams or jellies or try a regimen of proper diet and exercise. (We describe this in Chapter 6.) However, your health care practitioner may recommend hormone replacement therapy, arguing that nothing else will restore estrogen to the walls of the vagina and make them thicker and more resilient.

Vaginal estrogen creams are a form of hormone replacement designed to send the estrogen directly to the vagina. By applying the cream in much the same way you would use a contraceptive cream or jelly, you put the estrogen directly on the area where it is most needed. Unlike a contraceptive cream, however, you don't use the estrogen cream on an "as needed" basis but instead you follow a schedule devised by your practitioner. Because some estrogen is absorbed from the vaginal walls into the bloodstream, you will probably be advised to take progestin if you still have your uterus.

Vaginal cream may sound ideal if your only postmenopausal problem is atrophic vaginitis. However, these creams are not commonly prescribed, according to *American Druggist* (July 1993). Why not? Because estrogen doses depend upon how much cream you apply, doctors worry that you may not measure the cream precisely and thus take too little or too much estrogen—or that you may find the cream inconvenient to use and skip a few scheduled applications.

In addition, doctors talk about estrogen cream's unpredictable bioavailability—medicospeak for "we don't know how well your body absorbs estrogen from the vaginal walls." Doctors want to know exactly how much estrogen you're taking so that you take enough to make it work and so that you take the appropriate amount of progestin (if you still have your uterus) to counteract the dangers of unopposed estrogen.

So it's likely that if you are having painful sex or frequent vaginal infections, your practitioner will suggest HRT in pill or transdermal patch form. Because these problems are attributed to low levels of estrogen in your body, and stopping HRT would put estrogen at low levels again, the practitioner will probably recommend that you continue hormone replacement indefinitely so that similar problems don't recur.

Other genitourinary problems are related to the urinary tract. A need to urinate more frequently and recurring urinary tract infections are thought to be a result of low levels of estrogen after menopause. Just as reduced estrogen levels thin the tissues in the vagina, the tissues lining the urethra (the tube that drains urine from the bladder) become thin and more brittle. Again, your practitioner may recommend long-term hormone replacement—particularly in pill or patch form—to improve tissue elasticity.

Osteoporosis

Osteoporosis is a condition in which bones gradually lose their mineral content, becoming porous, thin and fragile. Causing pain, bone fractures (breaks) and loss of stature in its advanced stages, osteoporosis is one of the two greatest health hazards associated with menopause, according to the American College of Obstetricians and Gynecologists 1992

Technical Bulletin. The second hazard is heart disease, or cardiovascular disease, which we discuss later in this chapter.

Your bones are made of a combination of two types of tissue: **trabecular bone**, a porous bone tissue, and **cortical bone**, a dense and hard tissue. Flat bones and the vertebrae (backbones) are primarily trabecular bone surrounded by a thin layer of cortical tissue. Long bones such as the femur (thighbone) are primarily cortical tissue.

To varying degrees osteoporosis is a natural part of aging for both women and men. An adult's bones are at their peak density around age 35. After 40 bone mass slowly declines in men as well as women. Once a woman reaches menopause, however, the decline in bone mass continues at a much quicker pace. This accelerated phase lasts eight to 10 years, after which the bone loss slows to the pre-menopausal rate. In general women lose 50 percent of trabecular bone and 30 percent of cortical bone during their lives; men lose 30 percent of trabecular and 20 percent of cortical bone.

To determine your bone density, your health care practitioner will need to run one or more diagnostic tests, which include x-rays, photo absorptiometry scans and CT scans. (See "Measuring Bone Mass" on page 111 for the nuts and bolts of these tests.) It's not possible or accurate merely to "eyeball" a wrist, arm or leg to get an idea of how dense your bones are. The only clearly visible sign of bone loss is the curved back known as the dowager's hump, and by the time you can see this curve, you will have lost up to 50 percent of bone tissue in your vertebrae.

If your bones are strong to begin with, the gradual loss of bone tissue may not pose a problem in your old age. If your bones are thin in your 30s, then you run a greater risk of experiencing fractures at some time in your life. If your bone density is 20 to 30 percent lower than average, you have **osteopenia** (low bone mass). If your measurement is more than 30 percent lower than average, you have osteoporosis. Bone loss in the range of 30 to 40 percent can lead to fractures.

Fractures come in many forms, including **compression fractures** (breaks that collapse the bone, such as in the spine), **complete fractures** (breaks involving the entire width of a bone) and **incomplete fractures** (breaks that don't go all the way through a bone).

Why are fractures a concern? Fractures in the spine lead to stooped posture—the so-called dowager's hump. Fractures in the wrists can be inconvenient; those in the hips or legs can be incapacitating, necessitating surgery or prolonged medical care. The financial cost of treating fractures adds up: An estimated $7 billion is spent each year on acute and long-term care resulting from fractures. Fractures, particularly in the elderly, can be life-threatening: Five to 20 percent of older men and women who have a hip fracture die within 12 months of the injury—often from complications of hip surgery—and 15 to 25 percent are permanently disabled (*Current Obstetric and Gynecologic Diagnosis and Treatment*).

How Common Is Osteoporosis?

Twenty million women are affected by osteoporosis, according to 1990 figures from the National Osteoporosis Foundation. Each year approximately 800,000 American women develop fractures.

Some experts cite alarming statistics. Lila Nachtigall, M.D., an HRT advocate, writes in *Estrogen: The Facts Can*

Change Your Life that 93 percent of all American women who don't take estrogen will have a fracture in the arm, spine, hip or pelvis by age 85. She cites estimates that 25 to 35 percent of all women will eventually get severe enough osteoporosis to "cause them real trouble." (She does not define what she means by "real trouble.") Nachtigall also asserts that four out of 10 women show symptoms of osteoporosis. For that 40 percent she believes hormone replacement is essential.

Other experts say that the situation is less grim than those statistics suggest. Sheldon H. Cherry, M.D., and Carolyn D. Runowicz, M.D., authors of *The Menopause Book,* acknowledge that osteoporosis by definition is common, but that few women will be crippled by the disease— and that most women won't even know they have it. Cherry and Runowicz point to a study in which only 7 to 8 percent of the postmenopausal women examined were at high risk of fractures, while 20 percent were at intermediate risk and 70 percent at low risk. They state that "less than 10 percent of women over 70" have the kind of spinal fractures that could eventually lead to dowager's hump.

With such disparities in statistics, it's clear that you can't rely on the numbers to make your decision about taking HRT. You need to look at your own physique and medical history.

Osteoporosis: Are You at Risk?

Over the years researchers have found that certain factors indicate a tendency to develop osteoporosis. Which possible risk factors apply to you?

• Caucasian (particularly with a northern European heritage) or Asian race. According to *Current Obstetric and Gynecologic Diagnosis and Treatment,* osteoporosis occurs most often in Caucasians, then Asians, then African Americans.

• Slender or petite body frame

• Mother or father with osteopenia (low bone mass, a precursor of osteoporosis) or osteoporosis. A four-year study of hip fractures in Caucasian women, reported in the March 23, 1995, *New England Journal of Medicine,* suggests that you have double the usual risk of hip fractures if your mother had a hip fracture.

• Primary residence in northern areas of the country. More cases of osteoporosis develop in women in temperate climates than women in the tropics. This may be linked to the weak winter sun (sunlight on skin generates vitamin D, a necessary nutrient in maintaining bone strength) or to the fact that women get less outdoor exercise in the winter.

• Premature menopause or early surgical menopause not followed by a regimen of hormone replacement

• Late onset of menstruation (after age 16)

• History of irregular menstrual cycles

• History of **amenorrhea** (abnormal cessation of menstrual cycles)

• Diet low in calcium

• Cigarette smoking

• Excessive caffeine or alcohol intake. An article in the March 23, 1995, *New England Journal of Medicine* found that the more caffeine women consume, the higher their risk of fracturing a hip.

• Lack of exercise. A sedentary lifestyle is thought to promote bone loss. Postmenopausal women who spend fewer than four hours a day walking and moving around on their feet have double the risk of hip fractures than those who move around more, according to the *New England Journal of Medicine* article.

• Use of certain medications, such as steroids, anti-inflammatory medications, **sedatives** and thyroid hormones. These have been linked to osteoporosis or increased risk of hip fractures.

Okay, you've checked off any situations that apply to you. If you have one or more check marks, does this mean you will develop osteoporosis? Not necessarily. Nor do yes answers automatically mean you should start HRT—although some doctors rely on these risk lists in recommending hormone therapy.

A menopausal woman who is thought to be at risk should first be given an osteoporosis screening test. These bone density tests (see page 111), with fancy names like single-photon absorptiometry or computed tomography, give a snapshot of current bone thickness.

What will this test show? Well, it can show how you compare with a statistically average woman. If your bone mass is 20 percent lower than the average, the doctor sees cause for concern.

If the results show some bone loss, but less than 20 percent, then the case is less clear. In such a case, one test alone can't necessarily predict whether you're on the fast track to bone loss. Your doctor may want to perform another test in six months or a year to track changes in bone mass, estimate the rate of bone loss (remember, some bone loss is inevitable) and decide if steps need to be taken to slow the rate of loss.

In all cases a bone density test is most informative when compared against a **baseline**, which is the first test to which later ones are compared. In the context of bone health, the best baseline test would be one made in your mid- to late 30s, when your bones were at their strongest. Baseline bone density tests are not commonly taken that early in life. Instead doctors often have to perform a series of bone density tests over several months or years (depending on how slowly or quickly you lose bone mass) to get an accurate picture of how quickly your bone mass is changing. After age 40, cortical bone loss proceeds at .3 to .5 percent a year, increases to 2 to 3 percent for eight to 10 years during menopause, then returns to the slower rate. Trabecular bone has a shorter, but more accelerated, phase of bone loss, estimated at 4 to 8 percent a year, before it too slows.

Thus, if you are planning to take HRT solely to protect against the possibility of developing osteoporosis, you'd be wise to have your doctor order a bone density test before beginning therapy. Your bones may be strong and healthy, making hormone replacement unnecessary. In short, even though you may fit the "at risk" category, you may never develop osteoporosis.

The Osteoporosis-HRT Regimen

Let's say for the sake of discussion that you have a history of osteoporosis in your family and that several bone tests have confirmed rapid bone loss. Is HRT your only option? Not necessarily. A combination of weight-bearing exercise, vitamin D and calcium can stop bone loss (see Chapter 6), but this combination requires a disciplined commitment to nutrition and exercise. For the most part, the medical profession believes that few women want to make such a commitment or are disciplined enough to follow the necessary regimen. In its stead medicine offers

HRT. By taking estrogen, the theory goes, you can decrease your lifetime probability of experiencing an osteoporotic fracture.

Is HRT effective? The Food and Drug Administration (FDA) seems to think so: For a long time estrogen was the only drug approved by the FDA for use in preventing osteoporosis. (In October 1995 the drug maker Merck received clearance from the FDA to begin selling its Fosamax brand of alendronate for the treatment of osteoporosis.) The American College of Physicians claims that there is "limited but consistent evidence" that unopposed estrogen (estrogen without progestin) reduces the risk of hip fractures by about 25 percent and reduces the risk of spinal fractures by at least 50 percent. Combination therapy (estrogen with progestin) is assumed to offer the same protection, although the college admits that evidence to support this assumption is limited (*Annals of Internal Medicine,* December 15, 1992).

At the moment, the generally accepted approach for the prevention of osteoporosis, according to the American College of Obstetricians and Gynecologists, is a program of hormone replacement therapy, calcium supplements and exercise.

How much estrogen should you take to protect your bones? The current recommended range of estrogen doses (.625 mg to 1.25 mg of conjugated estrogen or its equivalent) for treating menopausal symptoms is also the amount of estrogen shown to guard against osteoporosis.

How Does Estrogen Protect Bone?

Scientists aren't exactly sure how estrogen halts bone loss, though they suspect that estrogen increases the bone's rigidity. Estrogen also preserves bone mineral and stimulates the thyroid gland's production of calcitonin (a hormone that stimulates bone production), and it may increase the body's ability to absorb calcium from the intestines.

However effective in stopping bone loss, estrogen and HRT cannot *rebuild* lost bone. For that reason some physicians push HRT use, opining that it "couldn't hurt" to protect yourself with estrogen supplements. Be aware that there are some practitioners who routinely prescribe HRT to prevent bone loss—even though some bone loss is normal in both men and women and even though not all women are at risk of developing osteoporosis.

If you decide to take preventive HRT, your practitioner will suggest beginning estrogen replacement within three years of your last menstrual period—and continuing it for life. That's because bone loss resumes once you stop taking estrogen, sometimes at that brisk pace associated with the first seven to 10 years after menopause.

In reality, however, you may tire of the cost of hormone medication, the extra doctor visits, and the possible side effects or risks. You may elect to take hormones for 10 to 20 years and then switch to a nondrug approach. Although bone loss will resume immediately after stopping hormones, it doesn't necessarily follow that you will develop osteoporosis immediately or, for that matter, ever. In taking estrogen for several years or decades, you may have at least temporarily slowed the clock on bone loss. That may be all you need to ensure a healthy, active life.

So what's the best strategy? Should you take HRT to prevent osteoporosis? It's true that estrogen has a crucial role in preserving bone tissue. If you are at high risk for osteoporosis, even the alternative therapies (e.g., diet and exercise) may not be enough to halt bone deterioration. But if your bone density is normal, then HRT may not improve it any further. You could possibly do yourself some harm in taking HRT unnecessarily. After all, the long-term risks of hormone replacement therapy have not yet been completely unearthed. (See Chapter 5.)

■ Measuring Bone Mass

By far the best way to determine if your bone mass is reaching dangerously low levels—levels that can lead to fractures—is through bone density tests. Here are some of the most common:

• **Radiographic absorptiometry (RA).** This is basically an x-ray taken of the hand to determine bone density, detect fractures and help the medical practitioner diagnose osteoporosis. X-rays are also occasionally taken to locate compression fractures and other types of fractures in the spine. The x-ray takes about three to five minutes to perform, but is less sensitive than the other tests listed next. They can't detect bone loss until 30 percent of bone mass has disappeared, so they are not the best method for detecting osteoporosis early.

• **Single-photon absorptiometry (SPA).** In this test, lasting about 15 minutes, radioactive iodine is used to determine the bone density of your wrist or heel. The radiation dose is about a tenth of that of the radiographic absorptiometry we just described. Radiation exposure is just a fraction of that of an arm x-ray and doesn't cost significantly more.

• **Dual-photon absorptiometry (DPA).** This test, also using radioactive iodine, measures the density of

▼

your spine, hip or thighbone. It exposes you to less radiation than the single-photon absorptiometry, lasts about 20 to 40 minutes and costs more than SPA.

• **Dual-energy x-ray absorptiometry (DEXA).** A DEXA scanner emits very low levels of x-ray radiation and a detector measures the amount of radiation absorbed by bone. The more radiation absorbed, the denser your bone. This test can be done on any part of your body—wrist, arm, spine, hip, thighbone—and is very quick (three to seven minutes). Although DEXA accurately measures the amount of bone tissue, it cannot detect fractures. The test usually costs more than the tests listed previously.

• **Quantitative computerized tomography (CT scans or QCT scans).** CT scans can measure trabecular bone within the vertebrae, the area where compression fractures occur, and create a 3-D image of your spine. But it does so with a much higher dosage of radiation than a DPA or DEXA. It also tends to overestimate the amount of bone tissue lost, critics charge. The scan takes 10 to 15 minutes and tends to be the most expensive of the tests listed here.

Your health care practitioner won't have all this equipment in the office, though he may be able to do the x-rays. Generally you'll be asked to visit a hospital or medical center to have these tests done.

Which test is best? Isaac Schiff, M.D., chief of the gynecology service at Massachusetts General Hospital, believes the best means of monitoring bone mass is with dual-energy x-ray absorptiometry done at the second bone of the vertebrae (located in the neck). This is "pre-

▼

cise enough to detect a loss or gain as little as 1 or 2 percent," he says in the January 1993 *Modern Medicine.*

What information can be gained from these tests? Bone density tests can show what your bones are like at a certain moment of time. When they are followed by later density tests, your doctor can get an idea of whether your bone density is increasing or decreasing, and at what rate. Individual measurements are usually compared with the average bone density of other women. If your measurement is 20 to 30 percent lower than average, you have osteopenia (low bone mass). If your measurement is more than 30 percent lower than average, you have osteoporosis. Bone loss in the range of 30 to 40 percent can lead to fractures in the spine and stooped posture.

Your practitioner may wish to supplement bone density tests with some tests geared to determining how quickly you are losing bone mass. One test, the **calcium to creatinine ratio**, is conducted on a urine sample taken first thing in the morning. A laboratory tests the sample for the ratio between calcium and a substance called creatinine. Because creatinine is produced at constant levels, changes in the ratio from the norm can indicate high calcium excretion suggesting bone loss. A high calcium intake (over 1,500 mg a day) can skew the results of this test.

A second test, called **urinary hydroxyproline**, also looks at calcium and creatinine and their ratio to an excreted substance called hydroxyproline, which can indicate bone loss. Because this test also detects the breakdown of other tissue, not just bone tissue, it doesn't always give an accurate picture of the rate of bone loss.

Heart Disease

Cardiovascular disease, or heart disease, as it's often called, is the leading cause of death in American women, according to the American College of Obstetricians and Gynecologists. Although heart disease is much more common in men than women under age 55, this difference begins to erode after 55. By the time women reach their 80s, they have the same incidence of heart disease as men.

Scientists believe that estrogen produced by the body gives women a protective advantage. They are not sure how estrogen protects the heart, but it's clear that estrogen increases levels of high-density lipoprotein (HDL, the so-called good cholesterol) and decreases levels of low-density lipoprotein (LDL, the "bad" cholesterol). In research conducted on animals, estrogen reduces the amount of fat (known as **lipids**) deposited on artery walls, decreases the amount of cholesterol deposited in blood vessels and increases the blood flow. Any of these might apply to humans and explain why estrogen seems to protect against heart disease.

Whatever the precise mechanism of estrogen on heart disease, scientists assert that one thing holds true: When ovarian estrogen declines after menopause, women lose their protective edge and gradually develop the same risk of coronary heart disease that men face.

A good deal of recent scientific evidence supports this hypothesis. The latest link in this chain of evidence was a carefully designed study of hormone replacement regimens published in the January 18, 1995, *Journal of the American Medical Association.* Conducted over three years at seven medical centers in the United States, the study followed 875 healthy women ages 45 to 64. The results showed that three HRT regimens—with or without progestin—all reduced women's risk of cardiovascular disease to some degree. The most beneficial regimen was unopposed estrogen (estrogen alone), a regimen that is not recommended for women who still have a uterus. The second most beneficial regimen was the combination of estrogen with 12 days each month of micronized progesterone (a little-known natural progesterone rarely prescribed by doctors). Less benefit was realized when conjugated estrogen (Premarin) was taken daily with the progestin medroxyprogesterone acetate (Provera). Although these results appear conclusive, the study's authors acknowledge that no one has yet shown that these lower risks actually translate into fewer heart attacks and strokes. In addition, the time span of the study was only three years—not long enough to gauge long-term impact.

Bernadine Healy, M.D., former director of the National Institutes of Health, noted in an accompanying editorial that it's not yet known how long women need to take HRT to get the maximum benefits and the lowest risks. Nor, she adds, has it been determined whether new methods of taking hormones, such as the transdermal patch, are as effective as taking estrogen orally.

Answers to questions about HRT's cardiovascular benefits and risks are one focus of the Women's Health Initiative, a long-term study now being conducted by the National Institutes of Health. Results of this study are not expected until sometime after the year 2000. For now the results from the January 18, 1995, *Journal of the American*

Medical Association article on the effectiveness of three HRT regimens is the most specific information about estrogen and heart disease to date. It underscores results of the Nurses' Health Study, a massive study of married registered nurses begun in 1976 and continuing today. Ten years of data on 48,470 postmenopausal women showed that those women taking estrogen were at significantly decreased risk for major coronary disease.

How much protection are we talking about? The American College of Physicians 1992 Clinical Guidelines for preventive hormone therapy states that "there is extensive and consistent evidence" that unopposed estrogen (estrogen given alone, without progestin) reduces the risk of heart disease by about 35 percent (*Annals of Internal Medicine,* December 15, 1992). Add progestin to the equation, as we mentioned before, and some of the benefit (but not all) disappears.

Heart Disease Risks

Menopause itself is presented as a heart disease risk. And the more years you live postmenopausally, without protective premenopausal levels of estrogen in your body, the greater this risk becomes.

But menopause is not the only risk for heart disease. Additional factors are at play:

• Mother or father who had a heart attack before age 55. If this is true for you, your risk of heart attack may be four or five times greater than average, say Cherry and Runowicz in *The Menopause Book.*

• Atherosclerosis. If you know you have heart disease (perhaps you've already had a heart attack), you are at greater risk.

- High blood pressure, such as a reading above 160/95
- Low HDL cholesterol levels and/or high LDL cholesterol levels
- Smoking. This increases risk even in young people, in part because it lowers HDL cholesterol.
- Diabetes. This disease results from the body's inability to produce or use insulin, resulting in high blood sugar levels. Diabetes can increase your risk of heart disease if it is not under control.
- Overweight. In particular, people who collect fat around the waist are at higher risk of heart disease than those who accumulate fat around the hips.
- Sedentary lifestyle
- Stress

No one disputes the importance of the above risk factors in predicting heart disease. But there is debate over whether menopause puts *all* women at risk of heart disease, or whether other risk factors must be present too. Kristen E. Smith, M.D., and Howard L. Judd, M.D., writing in *Current Obstetric and Gynecologic Diagnosis and Treatment,* report that "studies have suggested that the protective effect of estrogens on the heart is greatest in women with known risk factors for heart disease." In effect, we can, and should, question the wisdom of asking all menopausal women without contraindications to take HRT, when not all postmenopausal women are at risk of developing heart disease.

■ Risk Factors As Disease

In writing about cholesterol and heart disease in elderly Americans, *New York Times* medical reporter Gina Kolata pointed to a trend in modern medicine: the tendency of the medical profession to get all worked up about risk factors, to the point of treating people who have a risk factor for a disease with as much vehemence as if the people had the disease itself. But are practitioners treating the disease, or are they actually treating fear of the disease?

In her article Kolata examined the recent obsession with reducing cholesterol levels in the elderly. The reason for this obsession, she notes, is that high cholesterol levels are associated with an increased risk of heart disease. But high cholesterol levels are only a risk factor. Their presence does not guarantee that someone will have cardiovascular problems. In fact, some evidence suggests that people in their 70s and 80s have "dodged the heart disease bullet," and that high cholesterol levels at their ages do not pose a health hazard. Yet medical science continues to treat much of the elderly for high cholesterol.

"What has happened is that the risk factor has become the disease," said David Kritchevsky, M.D., a cholesterol researcher at the Wistar Institute in Philadelphia, in the pages of the November 2, 1994, *New York Times*. In Kolata's words, "High cholesterol levels themselves have come to be viewed as a pathology."

This "risk factors as disease" phenomenon can apply to hormone replacement therapy. One of the arguments for HRT today is that certain HRT therapies lower cho-

▼

lesterol levels. But does that mean fewer women will have heart attacks? Elizabeth Barrett-Connor, M.D., an author of numerous articles on hormone replacement, is one of several researchers who point out that it is not proven that cholesterol changes brought about by taking estrogen will reduce the number of heart attacks in post-menopausal women.

The lesson to you, the medical consumer, is to be sure that there are solid grounds for taking any drug therapy, be it something "natural" like estrogen or any other medication.

The Progestin Factor

In the past the addition of progestin to estrogen therapy was the big question mark in recommending preventive hormones for heart disease. Medical practitioners and concerned women alike wondered if progestin counteracted estrogen's probable protective benefits.

The latest research, as we mentioned earlier, suggests that progestin does indeed mute the benefits of estrogen alone, but that progestin does not completely cancel out estrogen's benefits. These results, however, have been based on short-term studies, and years will pass before we really know progestin's effect in the equation.

Until then, doctors still recommend progestin for women with a uterus to protect against the very real dangers of endometrial cancer posed by taking estrogen alone. (See Chapter 5.) If, given your heart disease risk, you decide that HRT is appropriate for you, the question then becomes what type of HRT to use.

As we mentioned earlier, research published in the *Journal of the American Medical Association* revealed that at least three regimens reduced women's risk of cardiovascular disease to some degree. The most beneficial regimen was unopposed estrogen (estrogen alone), a regimen that is not recommended for women who still have a uterus. The second most beneficial regimen was the combination of estrogen with 12 days each month of micronized progesterone (a little-known natural progesterone rarely prescribed by doctors). Less benefit was realized when conjugated estrogen (Premarin) was taken daily with the progestin medroxyprogesterone acetate (Provera).

The latter regimen (conjugated estrogen with medroxyprogesterone acetate) is currently one of the most commonly used regimens in the United States. If this regimen proves to be less beneficial to a woman desiring to lower her heart disease risk, she may wish to choose a less popular treatment option.

As to questions about the effectiveness of new methods of taking hormones, such as the transdermal patch, some data suggest that they may be less effective than estrogen. One researcher, Steven R. Cummings, M.D., of the University of California, San Francisco, claims that transdermal estrogen does not have the HDL-protective effect of oral estrogen. His findings, reported in *Family Practice News* (April 1, 1994), came from a computer analysis of data.

This doesn't mean you should remove transdermal patches from your list of options. Many women prefer the patch for its convenience; others, including those with a tendency to form gallstones or develop blood clots, choose the patch because that form of estrogen delivery is less likely to cause other health problems.

To date, the studies suggest that you need to continue taking estrogen to be protected against heart disease. Unless data show that there's an age beyond which HRT is no longer necessary, doctors will recommend long-term or lifelong hormone use for those women at risk of heart disease.

Where does this leave you? Your answer may depend on whether you and your doctor perceive you to be at risk of heart disease. If you've had past heart attacks, you may decide that hormone replacement therapy could prove lifesaving. If you are at low risk, your decision may be more difficult and may be influenced by your physician's point of view. Some practitioners promote HRT as a package deal: By taking it, they say, you can minimize menopausal symptoms, reduce the risk of osteoporosis and reduce the risk of heart disease. Other practitioners prefer to recommend HRT only for women at high risk—at least until all the data about estrogen and progestin's long-term adverse effects have been brought in. "As it stands today, postmenopausal women should not be taking hormones as the sole method of preventing heart disease," say Cherry and Runowicz in *The Menopause Book*. "Women should take other steps to prevent heart disease, with or without hormone therapy."

Stroke

Much of the medical literature explores estrogen's probable benefits to the heart (in particular, reduction of heart attacks). But researchers are also examining estrogen's role in preventing stroke—what doctors call a **cerebrovascular accident**. Strokes can cause weakness, temporary or permanent paralysis, even death. If postmenopausal estrogen replacement protects against coronary heart disease, researchers wondered, would HRT also protect against stroke?

Strokes can be caused by a hemorrhage (excessive bleeding) of a blood vessel in the brain or by a blood clot that blocks a blood vessel. Since a woman who has a history of abnormal blood clots is generally told not to take HRT, using hormones to reduce the risk of stroke seems to fly in the face of common sense. Nonetheless, several studies have looked at stroke-protective aspects of HRT. One study reported in the May 25, 1993, *Archives of Internal Medicine* examined data gathered from 23,088 women who took HRT three to six years. According to the studies' investigators, women who took 1 to 2 mg of estradiol compounds or .625 mg to 1.25 mg of conjugated estrogen at perimenopause (the years around the very last menstrual period) had a 30 percent lower risk of stroke than women in the general population who did not take HRT. The authors noted that the protective benefit of estrogen was mainly seen in women who continued to take the hormone, not in women who had stopped estrogen therapy.

Other studies dispute those findings. The Nurses' Health Study found no effect of postmenopausal estrogen use on stroke. And one landmark long-term study of heart disease, called the Framingham Study, reported in 1985 an increased risk of stroke among postmenopausal estrogen users, with women on estrogen 2.3 times more likely to suffer a stroke and 1.9 times more likely to develop heart disease than women who didn't take HRT. Since current research suggests that women on estrogen are less likely to develop heart disease, in contrast to the results of the Framingham Study, the link to increased risk of stroke is also being questioned.

Certainly more research needs to be done before HRT

can be recommended as a preventive therapy for stroke. Future study may contradict the data beginning to come out today. Just be aware that medical science continues to search for more uses for HRT.

Alzheimer's Disease and Other Memory Disorders

Connections are being explored between hormone replacement and memory lapses such as those occurring with Alzheimer's disease. The cause of Alzheimer's is unknown, but because the disease is more common in women than men (men are more likely to develop other forms of dementia), scientists are considering the possible connection of the hormone estrogen.

Victor Henderson and his colleagues from the University of Southern California presented findings to a 1993 meeting of the Society for Neuroscience suggesting that women on estrogen were 40 percent less likely to develop Alzheimer's than those who are not. While estrogen is clearly not the only factor contributing to the disease, Henderson and colleagues assert that hormone replacement may protect key cells in the brain, thus preventing or delaying the onset of dementia.

A few other studies have focused on the effect of estrogen use on verbal memory. In one recent assessment 71 healthy postmenopausal women took tests of their verbal and spatial memory, language skills, attention span and spatial skills. The scores of women taking estrogen were compared to those of non-users. The only significant differences were on tests of immediate and delayed paragraph recall, where women on estrogen scored much higher, leading researchers to postulate that estrogen affects verbal memory skills.

All this is preliminary research, and more needs to be done to determine whether a connection between estrogen and memory or Alzheimer's really exists.

Choosing Your Preventive Hormone Therapy

As you've seen, hormone replacement therapy can be taken to reduce genitourinary problems or to possibly protect against osteoporosis or heart disease. HRT may even be offered to you as a package deal—one that can protect you against all of those potential risks. The decision to take hormones is yours to make. The information in Chapters 5 and 6 is designed to help you make that very personal decision.

If you do decide to take long-term preventive hormone therapy, you'll be faced with several smaller but equally important choices. They include:

Taking estrogen alone (unopposed estrogen) or in an estrogen/progestin combination. Estrogen alone appears to offer stronger protection against heart disease. As we've discussed in previous chapters, estrogen alone (unopposed estrogen) is not recommended if you still have your uterus, because unopposed estrogen can lead to endometrial cancer. (See Chapter 5.) If you understand the risks, however, you can elect to use unopposed estrogen—provided you commit to physical exams once or twice a year and an annual endometrial biopsy to test your endometrium's health.

If you choose combination therapy, you can select estrogen and progestin in the cyclic therapy or estrogen and progestin in the continuous therapy. Current evidence suggests that the cyclic therapy offers better protection to the heart, while the continuous therapy is preferred by many women because it does not cause monthly menstrual-like bleeding.

Choosing your preferred form of estrogen. Depending upon what you hope to achieve with long-term therapy, you have the full range of HRT products to choose from. Most of the current research has focused on oral estrogen, so less is known about the effectiveness of patches, creams, injections and other new forms of estrogen distribution. (See Chapter 3.)

As we said before, research suggests that estrogen in pill form may give a better boost to HDL (good) cholesterol than the transdermal patch. However, if you can't take estrogen pills because health conditions contraindicate oral estrogen, then you may have to use the patch and know that it may be less effective in protecting against heart disease.

Deciding when to begin therapy. While hormone replacement can begin at any age during the menopausal process, most doctors suggest you make your decision soon after menopause—or at the time that your periods cease—advising you that HRT can slow down the otherwise rapid decline in bone mass during the first decade after your last menstrual period. Further, HRT is thought to protect best against heart disease when taken early.

Ensuring you get adequate medical care. Long-term hormone use requires a more diligent commitment to getting medical care. As with any drug, the longer you take hormones, the greater your chance of experiencing long-term side effects. (We'll discuss these in Chapter 5.) You'll need at least a yearly physical exam to monitor your health, and many doctors recommend one every six months. The Boston Women's Health Book Collective, writing in *The New Our Bodies, Ourselves,* recommends a checkup every three to six months.

In your checkups expect to receive breast and pelvic exams, a Pap smear, cholesterol and blood pressure tests, and annual mammograms if you're over age 50. If you still have a uterus and do not take progestin with your estrogen, you'll need an annual or twice-annual endometrial biopsy. (We discuss the elements of the physical exam in Chapter 3.)

Deciding how long to take hormones. Most HRT proponents believe that once you start preventive hormone therapy, you can (and should) take it for life to maintain its protective benefits. Health care practitioners who take a more conservative approach point out that you don't have to take it forever.

You may decide that osteoporosis is a risk, but a small one, so you may elect to protect yourself by taking extra estrogen only for five to 10 years; or you may feel that osteoporosis is a real hazard and elect to take HRT for 20 to 30 years.

You may feel that the expense and bother of medication, exams and annual tests are not worth the purported benefits of HRT and decide to stop it; or you may feel terrific on estrogen and decide to take it as long as possible.

More skeptical physicians believe that only women at high risk of heart disease and osteoporosis should take these drugs. And even the American College of Obstetricians and Gynecologists, whose 1992 Technical Bulletin tells physician-readers that HRT "can confer health benefits, enhance quality of life and prolong life expectancy," qualifies the statement by saying HRT is "not suited to all patients."

The truth of the matter is that no one really knows the effects of taking estrogen for 20 to 30 years. Studies involving low-dose estrogen, the type of estrogen thought to be safe today, only span 15 years, and many studies include data derived from women who used estrogen only.

In a sense, those of us who are taking HRT today are part of a large, real-life experiment. What the medical world learns from our experience will shape hormone replacement therapy as it is offered to future generations.

CHAPTER V

Long-Term Hormone Therapy: Issues of Risk and Safety

The arguments for taking hormone replacement therapy can be persuasive. Estrogen and progesterone, the argument goes, are natural substances produced by the female body, so why not take estrogen and progestin supplements once the body begins to reduce its production of these chemicals? There's no doubt that many women find the palliative and possible preventive benefits attractive reasons for taking hormone therapy. For a woman with debilitating hot flashes, the relief provided by hormones may be a boon and a blessing. A woman with a personal or family history of crippling osteoporosis may be relieved to find that HRT can protect against bone loss. Yes, estrogen and progestin are powerful drugs.

There's the rub! Estrogen and progestin are indeed drugs. And as medical consumers have repeatedly learned, every drug has side effects. In the short term, estrogen and progestin can cause water retention, bloating, breast tenderness, irritability, abdominal cramps and irregular, menstrual-like bleeding. (See Chapter 3 for a lengthy discussion of short-term side effects.)

The long-term risks associated with HRT are less clear. Although hormone replacement therapy has been around in some form for 50 years, the long-term hazards (if any) of taking HRT are matters of intense medical debate. At least one hazard, endometrial cancer, has been clearly linked to unopposed estrogen (estrogen taken alone, without progestin). Information on the impact of combination therapy (estrogen taken with progestin), the most popular form of HRT today, is just coming to light. Some of this information will not be released until the next century. What this means is that no clear evidence currently exists about how long-term HRT (therapy for 20 to 30 years) will affect your body.

What researchers and doctors have learned is that HRT can pose a danger to certain women. A woman usually is told not to take HRT if she has cancer of the breast, uterus or kidney (especially if the cancer is estrogen dependent—that is, it grows in the presence of estrogen); if she has had recent problems with blood clots in the major veins and arteries; if she has active liver disease or an impaired liver; or if she has any unexplained vaginal bleeding. These conditions are called absolute contraindications to HRT.

In other situations, taking HRT merits extra care and vigilance. If you have high blood pressure, gallbladder disease, diabetes, fibroids, migraines or endometriosis—all considered relative contraindications—your health should be monitored closely because HRT occasionally worsens these conditions. If that happens, you and your doctor may elect another form of estrogen (perhaps transdermal skin patches instead of pills) or decide to stop hormone replacement altogether.

If you have no absolute contraindications and none of the relative contraindications, does that make HRT safe? Many doctors will say yes, you can take it for life, as long as you get annual or semiannual medical physicals and develop no problems; other doctors will qualify that yes by saying that HRT is safe in the short term, but the verdict is not yet in on the effects of HRT taken longer than 10 years.

Why the lack of consensus between health care practitioners? For the complicated answer to that simple question, this chapter looks at what is currently known and unknown about long-term use of HRT and what that can mean to you.

Endometrial Cancer

According to 1987 figures from the National Cancer Institute, approximately 35,000 new cases of endometrial (uterine) cancer develop each year; about 2,900 women die from endometrial cancer annually. It is the third most common form of cancer in women.

A woman with a uterus who takes unopposed estrogen (estrogen alone) for 10 or more years has a four- to tenfold greater risk of developing endometrial cancer than women who do not take the hormone. And that increased risk persists for five to 15 years *after* you have stopped HRT, according to Elizabeth Barrett-Connor, M.D., of the University of California, writing in the *Annual Review of Medicine* (1992). However, says Barrett-Connor, endometrial cancer is usually caught early and thus generally has an excellent survival rate. But you wouldn't want to be the exception—nor would you want to develop cancer at all.

How does estrogen cause cancer?

To be precise, estrogen itself does not cause cancer. Estrogen promotes a dangerous, precancerous condition called **endometrial hyperplasia**—an excessive buildup or proliferation of cells that line the uterus. Here's how it happens: In your reproductive years estrogen thickens the lining of the uterus to prepare for a fertilized egg. If an egg is not fertilized, your body produces progesterone, causing the uterus to shed its tissue buildup. The result is menstruation. When estrogen is given after menopause, it also thickens the uterine lining. However, your ovaries are no longer releasing eggs and your body is no longer producing progesterone to initiate menstruation. Thus, the endometrial lining can continue to thicken. Eventually it may become so thick—over 4 mm—that hyperplasia develops.

Does all hyperplasia develop into cancer?

No. Hyperplasia can develop into cancer if it is neglected and if you are predisposed toward uterine cancer. A family history of endometrial cancer is a warning flag, as is obesity. (Women who are more than 20 percent over their proper weights are at a slightly greater risk of endometrial cancer. Their fat cells produce estrone, a form of estrogen; this means these women have greater amounts of estrogen in their bodies than women at or below their proper weights.) Other risk factors may include conditions such as diabetes, high cholesterol levels and high blood pressure.

However, the greatest risk factors appear to be the dose of estrogen you take and the duration of hormone therapy, according to the American College of Obstetricians and Gynecologists 1992 Technical Bulletin. The more unopposed estrogen you take, and the longer you take it, the greater your likelihood of developing hyperplasia.

What are the symptoms of hyperplasia?

Hyperplasia often causes unexpected (breakthrough) bleeding or unusually heavy or long-lasting bleeding. Be aware that hyperplasia can develop in the years before menopause, when your body's menstrual cycles become irregular and unpredictable. During the perimenopausal years hyperplasia causes very heavy menstrual periods and/or breakthrough bleeding. Unfortunately Pap smears do not always detect hyperplasia—a Pap test checks the health of the cervix outside the uterus, not the health of the endometrium. So every woman on estrogen must be alert to unusual bleeding such as heavy bleeding or spotting between scheduled periods, and inform her doctor. Tests such as an endometrial biopsy or a **dilatation and curettage** (**D&C**, a procedure in which the uterus is scraped clean) can determine if you have hyperplasia. (See "Evaluating the Endometrium" on page 136 for a closer look at these and other diagnostic tests.)

What can I do to protect myself against endometrial cancer?

To combat the dangers of unopposed estrogen, health care practitioners now prescribe progestin (a natural or synthetic progesterone) in tandem with estrogen for women with a uterus. Called combination therapy, the estrogen-progestin regimen has slowly gained a foothold as the HRT standard.

Progestin suppresses hyperplasia by preventing the thick uterine buildup. In rare cases hyperplasia can develop even if a woman is taking progestin—possibly because the woman is supersensitive to the effects of estrogen. Larger progestin doses may be needed. The key thing to remember is that women on combination therapy still need to pay attention to unusual bleeding.

How often do I need to take progestin to guard against hyperplasia and cancer?

Although no one yet knows the precise minimum number of days you need to take progestin to reduce the risk of endometrial cancer, studies suggest that most women are protected if they take at least 12 days of progestin each month.

How much progestin do I need to take?

If your HRT regimen calls for taking progestin for 12 to 14 days of the month, then the daily usual dose is 10 mg of medroxyprogesterone acetate. If you take progestin every day, the usual dose is 2.5 to 5 mg of medroxyprogesterone a day. These doses are really educated guesses. According to the American College of Obstetricians and Gynecologists, some research studies suggest that taking more than 12 days of 10 mg of progestin increases progestin's effectiveness. And when it comes to continuous therapy (taking progestin every day), not much data have been collected to show how effective continuous low-dose progestin is in protecting the uterus. This means that you may need a larger dose if you show signs of hyperplasia.

Is it ever possible to take unopposed estrogen?

As we mentioned earlier, unopposed estrogen is the treatment of choice if you have had a hysterectomy. However, if you have a uterus and take progestin and find that you cannot tolerate progestin's side effects (which can include bleeding, chronic headaches, nausea, cramps, irritability and depression), you can continue to take unopposed estrogen, but you *must* commit to annual tests (usually endometrial biopsies) to monitor the health of your endometrium. If the endometrium is found to be thicker than 4 mm, your health care practitioner may order additional procedures such as transvaginal ultrasound or a curettage. When it is caught early, treatment for hyperplasia usually consists of a two- or three-month course of progestin. This causes the uterus to completely and cleanly shed the built-up layer of cells in the endometrium, bringing the endometrium's thickness down to normal ranges. Hyperplasia is considered a potentially premalignant condition, which, left untreated, may develop into cancer. You *do* have the option of unopposed estrogen—but remember that you expose yourself to a four- to tenfold increase in cancer risk. Most doctors won't recommend that you take that risk.

According to the American College of Physicians Clinical Guidelines on HRT, "Women with a uterus have approximately a 20 percent lifetime probability of having a hysterectomy because of endometrial hyperplasia or cancer" caused by estrogen therapy (*Annals of Internal Medicine,* December 15, 1992). Hyperplasia is one of the most common reasons for hysterectomies—despite the fact that most early endometrial hyperplasia can be treated by taking two or three months of progestin, making surgery unnecessary.

As you would expect, estrogen shouldn't be taken if you have endometrial cancer. Nor should estrogen be taken if

(continued on page 138)

Evaluating the Endometrium

If your health care practitioner suspects you may be developing hyperplasia (a buildup of the tissue lining the uterus) or endometrial cancer, he will use one or more of the following tests to confirm his diagnosis:

• **Endometrial biopsy.** Also known as **endometrial sampling**, this is the standard method of evaluating the endometrium. A fairly simple and generally very accurate procedure, it is performed in a doctor's office. The practitioner inserts a narrow tube through the cervix into the uterus. Then a suction instrument or a cutting instrument (the latter is less common today) takes a sample of endometrial tissue and the tube is removed. The sample is examined by a pathologist under a microscope for signs of cancer. (A biopsy made by suction is sometimes called **aspiration endometrial biopsy**.)

An endometrial biopsy is performed every six to 12 months in women with a uterus who take unopposed estrogen. Annual biopsies are not thought to be necessary for women on estrogen-progestin therapy unless they have irregular bleeding.

• **Progesterone challenge test.** Instead of performing an endometrial biopsy, your health care practitioner may ask you to take progestin for 13 days to determine if you have an overly thick endometrium. If you bleed after stopping the progestin, the practitioner will take an endometrial biopsy to determine if you have hyperplasia or endometrial cancer. If you don't bleed, then it's unlikely that you have hyperplasia and an endometrial biopsy is not indicated.

Progesterone challenge tests may be given during the

▼

perimenopausal years if a woman's menstrual periods are irregular in flow and frequency. The purpose is the same as during premenopausal testing: to look for a buildup caused by too much estrogen stimulation in the uterus.

• **Ultrasound.** Sometimes an ultrasound (a picture of organs and structures deep inside the body made with high-frequency sound waves) is performed before a biopsy to determine whether you need tissue sampling. Your practitioner may order an abdominal ultrasound, in which a handheld probe is moved along the top of your abdomen, or a vaginal ultrasound, in which a narrow probe is placed into the vagina. In either case the probe emits ultrasonic waves which are used to measure the thickness of the endometrium.

Endometrial thickness greater than 4 mm is considered abnormal, and in such a case your practitioner will probably perform another test to take a tissue sample.

• **Hysteroscopy.** An endoscope (a flexible fiberoptic viewing tube) is inserted inside your uterus so your doctor can look at the endometrium and uterine walls. The doctor can use the tube to take a tissue sample of any areas that look unusual. This procedure can be performed in an outpatient clinic or in the hospital, and you'll probably be given an anesthetic.

• **Dilatation and curettage (D&C).** Performed as one-day surgery in the hospital or in a outpatient clinic, this medical procedure dilates (widens) the cervix so that the physician can scrape and remove the endometrium with a curette (a spoon-shaped instrument). Tissue samples are examined by a pathologist. D&Cs are performed for several reasons, including to investigate abnormalities found by an endometrial sample and to investigate abnormal and persistent bleeding. D&Cs are accurate but invasive, expensive and possibly painful. Further, you may have to be sedated or given anesthesia. D&Cs are no longer considered standard care for irregular bleeding. They have been replaced by hysteroscopies and aspiration endometrial biopsies for diagnosis.

you have an estrogen-dependent cancer such as some forms of breast cancer, because estrogen can accelerate cancer growth. Since you may not know if you have uterine or breast cancer, some doctors recommend that you have screening tests (an endometrial biopsy and a mammogram, for instance) done before beginning HRT.

If you have been successfully treated for stage I adenomatous hyperplasia (the very early stage of endometrial cancer), your practitioner may give the okay for HRT. Paul B. Marshburn, M.D., and Bruce R. Carr, M.D., professors of reproductive endocrinology at the University of Texas Southwestern Medical Center at Dallas, report that women with a history of stage I adenomatous hyperplasia "can receive estrogen replacement therapy without fear of disease recurrence" (*Postgraduate Medicine,* September 15, 1992). They state, however, that there are no long-term data on the safety of HRT in women who were treated for more advanced stages of endometrial cancer. For that reason a history of endometrial cancer is considered a contraindication to estrogen use.

How effective is progestin?

Several recent studies suggest that women who take a combined therapy of both estrogen and progestin have a lower incidence of hyperplasia or endometrial cancer than women who do not take HRT at all. That said, however, it must be noted that the long-term effects of progestin on the endometrium won't really be known for many years.

Breast Cancer

Approximately 10 percent of women will develop breast cancer at some time in their life. Some 175,000 to 180,000 cases of breast cancer are diagnosed in the United States each year, and 46,000 women die from this cancer annually. About three-quarters of breast cancers occur in women over age 44, during the perimenopausal and postmenopausal years.

What is the link between estrogen and breast cancer?

The possibility of a link between estrogen and breast cancer is an explosively controversial subject, to say the least.

On the one side of the debate are physicians who say that the vast body of scientific research—somewhere in the neighborhood of 30 studies—has found no conclusive connection between breast cancer and estrogen replacement. As Philip J. DiSaia, M.D., of the University of California, Irvine, School of Medicine, writes in a supplement to the journal *Cancer* (February 15, 1993), of the numerous studies attempting to evaluate the risk of developing breast cancer while on estrogen: "Most of these studies have not shown a significant increase in the incidence of breast cancer related to such therapy." The latest study that failed to find a link between breast cancer and HRT appeared in the July 12, 1995, *Journal of the American Medical Association*

(continued on page 141)

▌ Breast Cancer: What Is Your Risk?

You've heard the numbers: A woman has a one-in-eight chance of developing breast cancer—a statistic that has driven fear into the hearts of many women. The problem is you probably haven't heard the full story. When we talk about a one-in-eight risk, we're talking about the risk of developing cancer at the end of her lifetime.

In other words, at different ages women have different risks for developing breast cancer; as age increases, the risk for developing breast cancer rises. The National Cancer Institute Surveillance Program breaks down the numbers, specifying the varying risks for varying ages.

Age of a healthy, cancer-free woman	Risk of breast cancer
By age 25	1 in 19,608
By age 30	1 in 2,525
By age 40	1 in 217
By age 50	1 in 50
By age 60	1 in 24
By age 70	1 in 14
By age 80	1 in 10
By age 85	1 in 9
Ever	1 in 8

As you can see, the risk of developing breast cancer is far from negligible. But in the absence of other factors, your risk rises to a significant level only as you get up in years. Also, despite what you read elsewhere, remember that the risk of dying of breast cancer hasn't increased by a great deal in the last 20 years.

(JAMA). More than 1,000 women ages 50 to 64 (537 of them having had breast cancer diagnosed in 1988 through mid-1990) were surveyed about their estrogen and progestin use and their medical histories. The researchers "failed to find any increased risk of breast cancer associated with either current or long-term use of estrogen-progestin HRT." The *JAMA* article's authors note, however, that "the number of subjects who used this regimen for a long period is small, and subsequent studies will need to monitor the risk in those estrogen-progestin users who continue into their second decade of treatment."

On the other side of the estrogen/breast-cancer argument are those scientists and physicians who are uncomfortable with any increased cancer risk. They suspect an estrogen/breast-cancer link for many reasons: Breast cancer is much more common in women than men. Estrogen is known to affect breast tissue, occasionally encouraging abnormal cell growth and benign (harmless) cysts in the breasts (fibrocystic breast disease). Some forms of breast cancer are estrogen dependent, meaning they grow in the presence of estrogen. Then, too, extensive tests have shown that estrogens are associated with the development of breast tumors in animals.

While the association between estrogen use and breast cancer is hotly debated, there is new evidence that long-term use can increase risk to a statistically significant degree. A Harvard University study of long-term estrogen use, reported in the June 15, 1995, *New England Journal of Medicine,* found that women who took estrogen for five or more years after menopause had a 32 percent higher risk of breast cancer than women who had never taken the hormone. In those women who also took progestin, the risk was higher—41 percent. At greatest risk were women ages 60 to 64 who had used hormones five years or longer. They had a 71 percent higher risk of breast cancer than women who never took estrogen. The researchers also found that the risk of dying from breast cancer was 45 percent higher among estrogen users.

This Harvard study is significant in the number of participants—69,000 postmenopausal nurses who took part in the Nurses' Health Study from 1976 to 1992—and in the fact that the study examined all forms of HRT. The researchers found no difference in the effect of different forms of doses of estrogen.

Please remember, however, that these higher risks do not predict that most women on HRT will develop cancer. In fact, the study predicts that the actual percentage of women who will develop breast cancer in the next five years is still low. About 3 percent of 60-year-old women who have been taking estrogen for five years will develop breast cancer, compared to 1.8 percent of 60-year-old women not using hormones, Graham A. Colditz, lead author of the Harvard study, told the *Wall Street Journal* (June 15, 1995). Nonetheless, this greater percentage is enough to cause many women to reevaluate hormone replacement therapy. In the words of the Harvard study's authors, "These findings suggest that women over 55 years of age should carefully consider the risks and benefits of estrogen therapy, especially if they have used estrogen for five or more years. It is not clear that the benefits outweigh risks for all women, particularly women with few risk factors for heart disease." (As stated previously, one of the most persuasive arguments for HRT use today is the evidence that it can reduce heart disease—the number one killer of women—by 50 percent.)

Although the link between estrogen and breast cancer may seem conclusive, the medical establishment is awaiting the definitive answer on this issue. According to the National Institutes of Health (NIH), when all the results of the more than 30 studies of hormones and breast cancer are combined, "there is very little or no overall risk of breast cancer associated with the use of hormone replacement therapy." However, some studies suggest a risk associated with long-term hormone use, the NIH says.

Most physicians today believe that women who take low doses of estrogen (.625 mg or less of conjugated estrogen) run no increased risk of breast cancer. Some researchers suggest that the slight statistical increases in breast cancer revealed in several studies resulted not from the estrogen, but because the women on HRT were under closer medical supervision and thus their cancers were detected earlier and more often.

Are other risk factors associated with breast cancer?

Many experts assert that estrogen in and of itself doesn't cause breast cancer; they claim that other risk factors must be present. These factors heighten what doctors call the relative risk of breast cancer—relative meaning that the risk applies to a statistical sampling of women and may or may not apply to you in particular.

What are these breast cancer risk factors?

A family history of breast cancer; early onset of menstruation; late menopause; first childbirth after age 30; obesity; inactive lifestyle; smoking; and a high-fat diet are among the factors linked to breast cancer. Age is also a risk factor—the older you are, the more likely you are to develop this cancer.

In making the HRT decision, you and your doctor will want to weigh the possible increased risk of breast cancer with the possible cardiovascular and osteoporotic benefits of therapy. (We discussed these risks and benefits in Chapter 4.) More women suffer from heart disease than breast cancer. According to Daniel B. Williams, M.D., of Washington University School of Medicine, a woman's risk of dying from heart disease is 10 times greater than her risk of dying from breast cancer (*Internal Medicine News & Cardiology News,* September 1, 1994). Of course, this statistical risk refers to populations, not individuals. You are not a statistic, and your decision must reflect your own, highly personal concerns and risks.

Can I take HRT if I had breast cancer years ago?

For some women this question is a very real concern. Rena Vassilopoulou-Sellin, M.D., professor of medicine in the endocrinology section of the M. D. Anderson Cancer Center in Houston, surveyed 224 former breast cancer patients, 77 percent of whom were passing through menopause. "Of the menopausal women," Vassilopoulou-Sellin writes, "27 percent felt they needed some treatment for symptoms," while 70 percent were worried about the long-term menopause-related risk of osteoporosis and 72 percent worried about heart disease (*The Female Patient,* August 1993).

Everyone agrees that HRT is inappropriate for someone who is currently being treated for cancer. Medical experts disagree, however, about what is appropriate if you had cancer in the past. Philip DiSaia, M.D., acknowledges in the journal *Cancer* that "no prospective study has been conducted to test the impact of HRT on the survival of patients treated for breast cancer," but he states that there is "indirect proof" that "estrogen does not influence the outcome of patients with breast cancer." In the same vein, Vassilopoulou-Sellin in *The Female Patient* states that "the fear that estrogen promotes the growth of breast cancer remains unsubstantiated," and concludes that "previously extant breast cancer should only be considered a relative contraindication to the prescription of estrogen replacement therapy that is otherwise indicated."

The implication is that if you have been successfully treated for breast cancer, and you want to take HRT to ease your menopausal symptoms or to guard against osteoporosis and heart disease, then you should be able to take it—being aware that "freedom from recurrent breast cancer can never be guaranteed," according to DiSaia.

But many doctors are uncomfortable recommending HRT when its safety and benefit for successfully treated breast cancer patients have not been tested in controlled clinical trials. In light of the difficulty in ascertaining that no dormant cancer remains in a woman's body, how does one define the cured or successfully treated cancer survivor? This is a concern of Douglas J. Marchant, M.D., of the Breast Health Center at Women and Infants Hospital in Providence, Rhode Island. He writes in the March 15, 1993, *Cancer* supplement, "Given the uncertainty about hormone interactions and the molecular genetics of breast cancer, it seems unwise to inject yet another element into the prognostic equation." He does not recommend that HRT be used routinely in women who have been treated for breast cancer, although he acknowledges that the final decision rests with a woman, her family physician and her oncologist.

Your practitioner will have a personal point of view. The doctor may argue against HRT for women who have had cancer; or may suggest it for a very brief period to relieve extremely severe menopausal symptoms; or may agree that it is useful, under careful medical supervision, for women who have had cancer but are also at high risk of osteoporosis or heart disease. If you have had breast cancer and are weighing HRT use, it would be wise to get at least one other opinion from a highly reputable cancer specialist or cancer center.

Some doctors state that estrogen can decrease the size of non-estrogen-dependent tumors, especially if the estrogen is combined with progestin. Many doctors today recommend that their patients on HRT take progestin—even if a woman has no uterus—arguing that progestin may protect against breast cancer. At the moment, this is experimental, even speculative, treatment. While one research study has reported that progestin protects against breast cancer, other investigations have claimed no effect, and still others report an increased cancer risk when progestin is added to estrogen therapy. Be aware that the only currently approved rationale for adding progestin to HRT, according to the American College of Physicians 1992 Clinical Guidelines, is for guarding against endometrial cancer.

The role of both progestin and estrogen in breast cancer should be clearer in future years as HRT is investigated more thoroughly in clinical studies. Until then the impact of HRT on breast cancer remains unclear.

Thromboembolic Disease

Thromboembolic disease refers to a medical condition in which people develop blood clots that block blood vessels. A blood clot is known in scientific lingo as a **thrombus** or an **embolus** (although *embolus* can also refer to an object or a bit of tissue or gas in a blood vessel). When a thrombus forms in a blood vessel, the condition is known as thrombosis. When an embolus blocks a blood vessel, it is called an **embolism**.

Whatever the name, blood clots are a major cause of heart attacks and strokes. Blood clots in an artery supplying the brain cause a stroke; clots in an artery supplying the heart cause a heart attack; blood clots in a vein cause an inflammation of the vein known as thrombophlebitis, which is one of the causes of varicose veins. Thrombophlebitis can be dangerous. The blood clot can break away from the wall of the blood vessel and travel to the heart, causing a heart attack.

What is the connection between estrogen and blood clots?

The general consensus today is that HRT poses a risk only for the woman who has a pronounced history of thromboembolic disease or who has recently had a blood clot. Thrombophlebitis is considered a relative contraindication—meaning that in some cases, and with attentive medical care, a woman with thrombophlebitis could take HRT. Varicose veins (which can be caused by weak or defective valves in a vein, by pregnancy or by obesity) are not a contraindication.

Why is HRT a problem for women with thromboembolic disease?

The answer appears to lie in the way estrogen affects the liver. Estrogen encourages the liver to produce some substances called clotting factors while suppressing the production of some anticlotting factors. This is usually not a problem for most women on the low doses of estrogen, especially conjugated estrogens, used in HRT today (although it can be a problem for women who take estrogen at high doses, such as in some birth control pills). Additionally research some years ago showed an increased risk of blood clots in postmenopausal women using synthetic estrogens (in particular, ethinyl estradiol and mestranol), according to Wulf H. Utian, M.D., writing in *Managing Your Menopause*. Today's estrogen of choice is conjugated estrogen, one of the natural estrogens sold on the market.

However, if you have a history of heart attack, heart failure or stroke, or if you've recently had blood clots, then your liver might be producing clotting factors and suppressing the production of some anticlotting factors. HRT should be used with great caution, if at all. If you develop thrombosis or embolism, then hormone replacement therapy should be discontinued, according to the American College of Obstetricians and Gynecologists 1992 Technical Bulletin.

Are there other risk factors associated with blood clots?

As with any medical condition, certain preexisting conditions put any woman at greater risk of developing blood clots, including a history of blood clotting, smoking, obesity and severe varicose veins.

Is there any way to protect against blood clotting?

Since oral estrogens can alter the blood's clotting substances slightly, many experts now recommend other HRT regimens (such as the skin patch) because they apparently leave the clotting factors unchanged. A computer analysis of the benefits and risks of HRT by Steven R. Cummings, M.D., of the University of California, San Francisco, buttressed the recommendation that transdermal estrogen is the form of choice for women with thromboembolic disease (*Family Practice News,* April 1, 1994).

Another way to protect against blood clotting is to take aspirin regularly—one-half to one aspirin taken every two or three days. (Check with your practitioner for specific doses.) Scientists suspect that aspirin keeps small cells in the blood (**platelets**) from lumping together and forming clots. No clots, no heart attack or stroke. A large national study reported in the *Annals of Internal Medicine* in mid-1991 concluded that alternate-day, low-dosage aspirin therapy greatly reduces the risk of a first heart attack among people with chronic stable angina—a group at high risk for cardiovascular disease. And in findings presented at the annual meeting of the American College of Cardiology in 1991, researchers at Oxford University in England underscored the results of more than 200 studies of aspirin. These studies, said the Oxford team, provide conclusive evidence that aspirin can cut the risk of a second heart attack or stroke by 25 percent. Clearly the role of aspirin in preventing blood clots is an issue to discuss with your health care practitioner.

Hepatic Effects

The term *hepatic* refers to the workings of the liver, a large gland found in the upper right of your abdominal cavity. The liver has many important jobs, among them secreting the thick fluid bile (sometimes called **gall**), producing blood-clotting substances, regulating blood sugar levels and neutralizing poisonous substances. The liver works in association with the gallbladder, a reservoir for bile located on the lower side of the liver. Bile produced in the liver passes through the hepatic duct to the gallbladder, which stores the bile until it is needed by the small intestine to break down fatty foods.

How does HRT affect the hepatic system?

Research suggests that women on estrogen are two and one-half times more likely to develop gallstones. The risk increases if you are obese (more than 20 percent over your ideal weight). The American College of Obstetricians and Gynecologists lists active liver disease and chronic (long-lasting) impaired liver function as contraindications to estrogen replacement therapy.

What does estrogen do to the liver and gallbladder?

Estrogen can affect them in several ways. When estrogen is taken orally (in pill form), it is processed by the liver before it goes into the bloodstream. An impaired or diseased liver may not properly convert estrogen; in turn the estrogen may become a toxin in the body. Many doctors believe that the hormones in vaginal estrogen creams and transdermal patches are safe because they are not taken orally and thus the estrogen bypasses the liver.

Estrogen, particularly oral estrogen, also increases the odds of developing gallbladder disease. Estrogen encourages increased amounts of cholesterol to collect in the bile manufactured by the liver. The bile becomes supersaturated with cholesterol, and gallstones (three-quarters of which are composed primarily of cholesterol) form. These stones are often painful and sometimes must be removed by surgery.

Estrogen in the form of pills and tablets is usually off-limits to women with gallbladder problems. Transdermal patches and vaginal creams are thought to be safe options because the estrogen is absorbed into the bloodstream through the skin and doesn't pass through the liver. Be aware, however, that clinical studies haven't determined whether patches actually reduce the incidence of gallstones. If you have a history of gallbladder disease or gallstones and you choose to try HRT, be sure your doctor monitors the effects of therapy on your body. If you develop gallstones during the course of HRT, then you should reevaluate your treatment regimen and perhaps change your diet (such as reducing cholesterol). Switching from an oral estrogen to a skin patch may be an option—although, again, no clinical studies confirm the effect of patches on gallstones.

Other Possible Effects

As hormone use comes under closer scrutiny, researchers unearth other possible connections between hormone replacement therapy and other health conditions. Some of these include:

• **Hypertension (high blood pressure).** Oral contraceptives, with their high doses of estrogen, are known to increase the risk of high blood pressure. So naturally the medical profession has carefully watched HRT for similar problems. Some doctors believe that HRT may provoke high blood pressure or make an already existing hypertension worse, "but most evidence shows no such causal relationship," according to education and counseling guidelines published in the October 1990 *Journal of Gerontological Nursing.*

Because there are occasional reports of unusual cases of hypertension ascribed to HRT, the journal advises its nurse readers to take blood pressure measurements shortly after a woman starts hormone replacement and to check blood pressure levels regularly while the woman is on hormones. An article in *Drug Topics* (February 5, 1990) suggests that those women who experience elevated blood pressure from oral estrogen might not have this problem with the transdermal patch. That said, high blood pressure is considered a relative contraindication for HRT, which means that if you have hypertension, your doctor should monitor your therapy carefully.

• **Ovarian cancer.** The possibility of a link between HRT and ovarian cancer—a particularly devastating cancer because it rarely shows symptoms until it is in an advanced stage—was raised by Elizabeth Barrett-Connor in the *Annual Review of Medicine* (1992). Although she notes that at least 10 case-control studies were unable to link ovarian cancer with HRT, some studies from Britain have revealed areas of concern. One study found a 2.5-fold increase in ovarian cancer risk, with the highest risk associated with high doses of all types of estrogen. Another study found an increase in cancer over time, with an estimated risk of 1.7 for five to nine years of estrogen therapy and 2.4 for 10 or more years of therapy. Barrett-Connor believes it may be "premature to exonerate hormone replacement as a risk for ovarian cancer."

• **Eye problems.** The transdermal patch is a relatively new product, and some problems are coming to light as more women use it. In particular, some women who use estrogen patches after a **total hysterectomy** experience eye problems such as blurred or fluctuating vision; dry, itchy, burning, watery eyes; pain in the eye, or a pulling sensation within the eye, according to Andrew Gurwood, O.D., and his colleagues from the Pennsylvania College of Optometry, writing in the January 1995 *Optometry and Vision Science.* See your physician or ophthalmologist if you have such eye problems while using HRT. If underlying eye health problems are ruled out by your practitioner, the doctor may want to consult with your gynecologist about switching from the patch to another form of estrogen, Gurwood and colleagues observe.

Stopping Hormone Therapy

How long should you stay on HRT? The answer depends upon what you wish to achieve:

• If you simply wish for relief from menopausal symptoms such as hot flashes, most doctors advise two to five years of therapy.

• If you want to protect yourself against osteoporosis and heart disease, but are concerned about the risks of long-term HRT, your practitioner may suggest seven to 10 years of therapy. While the bone- and heart-protective qualities of HRT quickly diminish once you stop therapy, you will have gained seven to 10 years' worth of protection (which may be all you need if you are at low risk).

• If you are extremely concerned about or at high risk of osteoporosis and heart disease, and you want lifelong protection against vaginal atrophy and urinary tract infections, your practitioner may suggest taking hormones for as long as you live. Keep in mind, however, that lifelong HRT still falls into the category of unproved or controversial therapies.

Naturally all these therapies hinge on your not having contraindications or developing dangerous side effects such as hyperplasia.

How many women take HRT? About 11 million women a year. Anywhere from 12 to 32 percent of postmenopausal women are "current users" of hormone replacement therapy, according to a review of recent medical surveys by Erin K. Scalley, B.S., and Janet B. Henrich, M.D., of the Yale University School of Medicine (*Journal of Women's Health,* Fall 1993). That number of current users is smaller than doctors think. Studies have found that only 15 to 50 percent of women who are prescribed oral estrogen actually take their medication, note Scalley and Henrich. In contrast, women who use the transdermal patch comply with their HRT regimens 95 percent of the time.

Among women who are currently taking hormones, fewer than a quarter of them take estrogen with progestin, Scalley and Henrich report. Most women take unopposed, low-dose (.625 mg) oral conjugated estrogen—and they take it for two years or less.

Why do so few women continue HRT? The reasons, Scalley and Henrich write, are "improvement in their symptoms or, conversely, a lack of improvement; forgetfulness; and difficulty with complex regimens." Side effects, such as cyclic bleeding and breast tenderness, and concerns about safety were also common causes.

Some women stop HRT under the direction of their physician; some decide they are ready to quit and their practitioners concur with the decision. You may decide to stop therapy for any of a variety of reasons:

• You cannot cope with the return of monthly bleeding (periods). (This is frequently cited as the number one reason women stop HRT.)

• You have been taking short-term HRT to relieve menopausal symptoms, and two to five years have passed, making the time right to phase off hormones.

• You have tried HRT but found you disliked the short-term side effects like painful breasts.

• You dislike the inconvenience of taking pills and having extra physical exams and tests and their costs.

• You have discovered that you have a medical condition that contraindicates hormone therapy.

• New evidence has come out about some health hazards associated with HRT, and you have decided that you don't want to put yourself at risk.

These are all legitimate reasons to talk with your practitioner about discontinuing hormone therapy.

What is worrisome to the medical profession is noncompliance—that is, women who receive prescriptions and never have them filled, or who start therapy and then stop taking the hormones, or who take hormones sporadically, or who should be taking estrogen and progestin but skip the progestin part.

The problem with noncompliance is not so much that

women don't take HRT (although naturally that is a concern), it's that they may not tell their practitioners that they've stopped therapy.

This is not to suggest that you should take HRT against your will or against your better judgment. But for many reasons you should tell your practitioner if you decide not to continue HRT. Your practitioner may assume that you are taking hormones and may adjust other medications to suit. He may attribute some improvement in your health (such as a slowing in the progression of osteoporosis) to your taking HRT, when in fact the success may be due to something else. If you wish to stop estrogen and/or progestin, your practitioner may be able to recommend alternative therapies to HRT. But you won't find out unless you are up-front and open.

In fact, if you don't feel that you can be honest with your health care practitioner and talk about your attitude toward HRT, then it's time to find a new physician. Find someone with whom you can communicate; be an active medical participant in your health care.

How to Discontinue HRT

Your practitioner can guide you in setting up a plan to discontinue hormone therapy, depending in part on what form of estrogen you are taking (pill, patch, cream), how much of it you take and how much progestin (if any). In general the strategy is to taper off gradually. An abrupt cut-off can put you into full-fledged estrogen withdrawal, complete with severe menopausal symptoms like hot flashes—the very thing many women take HRT to avoid. These occur for the same reason that original menopause symptoms occur—a sudden and sharp drop in estrogen levels.

Some women experience hot flashes even if they gradually phase off HRT. These symptoms are usually temporary. Thus, in the same way that you and your doctor had to fine-tune your estrogen-progestin doses when you started HRT, some adjusting of hormones may be needed as you taper off.

Your doctor may suggest slowing the frequency of taking estrogen, recommending that you take it every second or third day. Or he may prescribe a smaller dose or ask you to halve or quarter the estrogen pill. A patch can be cut into smaller pieces and applied as usual. It may take your body three or four months to adjust to the declining estrogen levels.

If you have been taking progestin, you'll probably be told to continue the progestin at the usual level until you are finished with the estrogen. Why not cut back the progestin immediately? Because as long as you're taking estrogen, you'll need to guard against hyperplasia, a precancerous buildup of the uterine lining. In Britain, where women can choose to get estrogen through skin implants, progestin may be given a year or more after a woman has stopped using estrogen implants, because estrogen can stimulate the endometrium for up to two years after the last implant, according to a February 1, 1992, *Lancet* article.

Can you resume HRT? In most cases, yes. If you decide you want the possible long-term protection for heart disease and osteoporosis, you can almost always restart hormone therapy at a later date, under the guidance of your physician.

What's Next?

So far in this book we've looked at the short-term and long-term protective benefits of hormone replacement therapy. And we've explored the known and unknown risks. But to make a fully informed decision about trying HRT yourself, you need another piece of the puzzle: information about alternatives to hormone replacement therapy—things you can do before starting HRT, instead of HRT or during HRT. We look at these next.

. . . .

CHAPTER VI

Alternatives and Adjuncts to HRT

H ormone replacement therapy's benefits, HRT's risks. By the time you've reached this chapter, you have a pretty solid picture of the pros and cons of hormone replacement. You may have made a tentative decision about whether HRT is right for you. But before you open (or close) the door to hormone replacement, look closely at the alternatives.

For a woman in menopause or postmenopause, HRT is one tool to cope with the discomforts and guard against conditions such as osteoporosis and heart disease. And while this tool may be the current favorite of mainstream medicine, it is not the only tool available. For women who cannot or do not want to use estrogen, alternatives exist.

Writing in the December 1993 *American Journal of Public Health,* Lynn Rosenberg, Sc.D., states that "hormone supplements are being proposed as a preventive of conditions for which alternative methods of prevention are known and feasible." Women at increased risk of heart disease, she says, can take blood-pressure-lowering drugs and lose weight if they have high blood pressure, or they can change their diets or take cholesterol-lowering drugs if they have high cholesterol levels. Options exist for women at increased risk of osteoporosis, Rosenberg states.

Her point is that the American medical system is too quick to prescribe hormone replacement for too broad a spectrum of women—especially since other, sometimes nonpharmaceutical steps can be as effective in lowering a woman's risk of what are portrayed as menopause-related health conditions. These skeptics note that hormone replacement is unnecessary for all but those women at very high risk of osteoporosis or heart disease.

Many HRT proponents will argue in turn that these steps can be seen as *adjuncts* to hormone replacement— steps that will make estrogen work more efficiently at improving a woman's health.

To help you judge the merit of these arguments—and to help you make an informed decision about HRT—this chapter explores the most common alternatives and adjuncts to hormone replacement.

We begin by talking about pharmaceutical alternatives to estrogen. Then we'll look at lifestyle changes that some experts claim can be as effective as HRT. Finally we'll examine alternative medicine, such as homeopathy, herbal medicine and **biofeedback**, that some women find valuable in making their life healthier during and after menopause.

Pharmaceutical Alternatives to Estrogen

Hormone replacement therapy is often recommended to women to treat a number of menopausal and postmenopausal problems, including hot flashes and long-term health conditions such as heart disease and osteoporosis. However, other drugs exist that can address menopausal discomforts and menopause-related health conditions separately.

Medications for Hot Flashes

PROGESTIN

Progestin may be an option for women who want relief from hot flashes but don't want to take estrogen. In this case the physician will usually prescribe a low dose (2.5 mg a day) of medroxyprogesterone acetate in pill form.

A synthetic progestin known as megestrol acetate (Megace) is used to give relief to pain and other symptoms associated with advanced breast or endometrial cancer. It can help control hot flashes in women who have had cancer.

Progestin does not work for all women, however. Most mainstream medical practitioners believe estrogen is more effective for more women. When progestin does work, it starts providing relief in two to three weeks, with the best results achieved after a month or so of therapy. The higher the dose, the greater the relief. Higher doses, however, can lead to progestin-related side effects, such as breakthrough bleeding, water retention and bloating, breast swelling and tenderness, weight gain and depression and irritability. (See Chapter 3.)

If you have endometriosis or cancer and cannot take estrogen, but you are experiencing hot flashes, your doctor may administer a long-acting form of medroxyprogesterone acetate that is injected under the skin or into a muscle every two or three months. This form of progestin is not FDA-approved for treating menopausal discomforts, although it may be used in the treatment of endometriosis or cancer.

Although your practitioner would not prescribe this injected progestin just to treat hot flashes, in some women relief from hot flashes is a side effect of this drug. Its drawback is unpredictable withdrawal bleeding. (In contrast, withdrawal bleeding with progestin in pill form is usually extremely predictable.)

ANTIHYPERTENSIVES

These medications used to lower blood pressure can relieve hot flashes. While your doctor would not prescribe an **antihypertensive** medication if your blood pressure is normal, these drugs are an option for menopausal women with elevated blood pressure who want relief from hot flashes.

One of these medications is **clonidine**, sold as Catapres and in generic form. It appears to reduce the frequency of menopausal symptoms by stabilizing the body's thermostat. Clonidine's most common side effects are dry mouth and drowsiness, occurring in a third of women using it. Constipation, weakness and insomnia are also reported effects.

Methyldopa (sold as Aldomet and in generic forms) is another blood pressure medication that reduces hot flashes. Side effects are less common with methyldopa and generally occur just at the start of treatment, according to the *Physicians' Desk Reference.* These side effects include dry mouth, headache, weakness and fatigue.

SEDATIVES AND TRANQUILIZERS

Sedatives decrease activity, relieve anxiety and calm a person. They can have general, overall effects, or they can affect certain organs (such as the vasomotor system, the part of the nervous system that controls the narrowing and widening of the blood vessels). **Tranquilizers** also have a calming effect, lessening anxiety and tension and inducing drowsiness. Some tranquilizers can reduce muscle spasm. Both sedatives and tranquilizers are prescribed, albeit infrequently, to relieve hot flashes.

Sedatives can allay menopausal discomforts such as hot flashes and drenching sweats through their effects on the nervous system. One popular sedative for this purpose is Bellergal-S, an antispasmodic drug used to treat palpitations, "nervous stomach" and vasomotor disturbances such as hot flashes, sweats, restlessness and insomnia. Bellergal's side effects—for example, dry mouth, constipation, tingling in the hands and feet and blurred vision—occur rarely, according to the *Physicians' Desk Reference.* However, it contains phenobarbital, a chemical that can be habit-forming. Some doctors argue that phenobarbital levels are low in Bellergal-S, thus making it safe to take. But other doctors are uncomfortable prescribing any drug—tranquilizer or sedative—that may be addictive when other medications to treat hot flashes are available.

In similar fashion the tranquilizers chlordiazepoxide (Librium) and diazepam (Valium) are sometimes prescribed to women who experience hot flashes, anxiety, irritability and mood swings during menopause. Librium reduces anxiety in ways scientists don't yet understand; Valium affects the hypothalamus, that part of the brain that controls the body's thermostat, as well as the endocrine system and parts of the nervous system. Both of these drugs are highly addictive and should be used for as short a time as possible. The *Physicians' Desk Reference* suggests short-term use—less than four months. Side effects can include drowsiness, weakness and fatigue; and withdrawal symptoms such as vomiting and cramping can occur if the drug is abruptly discontinued.

Medications for Osteoporosis

SALMON CALCITONIN

Commonly called calcitonin and sold as the brand names Calcimar and Miacalcin, **salmon calcitonin** is approved by the Food and Drug Administration to prevent further bone loss in women who already have osteoporosis. Like estrogen, salmon calcitonin cannot reverse bone loss, but it can prevent further deterioration.

There are three drawbacks to calcitonin therapy as currently available in the United States. First, it is very expensive: A year's therapy costs about $3,600, according to the 1995 *Merck Manual.* Second, calcitonin must be injected, which many women find inconvenient and unpleasant. Third, the therapy may become less effective over time. According to a July 1993 article in *American Druggist,* the body may develop calcitonin antibodies from long-term use, reducing (but not negating) the therapy's effectiveness. Side effects of calcitonin therapy, according to the *Physicians' Desk Reference,* include nausea and redness or swelling at the site of injection.

Just as *The Hormone Replacement Handbook* was going to press in late 1995, a nasal-spray version of salmon calcitonin was approved for use in the United States by the Food and Drug Administration. According to research so far, this version is purer than the injected calcitonin, leading scientists to postulate that it will be less likely to raise calcitonin antibodies. Whether the nasal spray will prove to be less expensive than the calcitonin injection remains to be seen.

In either case women with allergies to salmon could be allergic to either form of this medication. You should have a skin test done in an allergist's office before taking calcitonin for the first time. In some cases it could cause a severe, life-threatening allergic reaction.

BIPHOSPHONATES

This class of drugs can also prevent further bone loss, but **biphosphonates** are not approved by the Food and Drug Administration for this use. (Biphosphonates are used to treat bone cancer.) They work by reducing **bone resorption**, the process by which the body removes calcium from bones. Frequently prescribed to treat **Paget's disease** (a bone disease characterized by excessive bone destruction and poor bone structure, which can lead to bone pain, frequent fractures and skeletal deformities), these biphosphonates can also be used to stop the progression of osteoporosis.

Etidronate (Didronel) and **pamidronate** are two biphosphonates that are injected into the body. Etidronate is also available in pill form and appears to prevent and treat osteoporosis of the spine. For biphosphonates to work effectively, adequate amounts of calcium and vitamin D must also be taken, says the 1995 *Merck Manual. American Druggist* describes the ideal regimen as a cycle of two weeks of etidronate pills followed by 11 to 13 weeks of calcium. Side effects of etidronate include diarrhea and nausea.

CALCITRIOL

This drug, generally prescribed to people with severe kidney disease, is new to the osteoporosis arsenal, according to Sadja Greenwood, M.D., author of *Menopause, Naturally.* An active form of vitamin D in the body, calcitriol appears to be an effective osteoporosis medicine, at least according to preliminary studies. However, Greenwood writes, overdoses of this drug can cause kidney stones. If you and your doctor choose this new medication, you should monitor yourself for this side effect.

SODIUM FLUORIDE

Once a mainstay of treatment for advanced osteoporosis and widely used for over 30 years, this drug has fallen out of favor. Studies suggest that while sodium fluoride increases bone density in women who take it, it doesn't reduce the number of fractures women ultimately experience. So even though this drug was once widely used, the American College of Obstetricians and Gynecologists considers sodium fluoride use to treat osteoporosis experimental.

Medications for Vaginal Dryness

Vaginal lubricants are pharmaceutical products that can be purchased over the counter or acquired through a physician's prescription. The lubricants counter vaginal dryness, which can lead to uncomfortable or painful sexual intercourse.

Water-based lubricants (such as K-Y Jelly or Gyne-Mostrin Gel) and vaginal suppositories (Lubrin Vaginal Lubricating Inserts) soothe a dry vaginal wall for several hours. They can be applied as often as needed, generally before intercourse.

A moisturizing gel called Replens reputedly gives longer relief, as each application lasts two to three days. Touted as the next best thing to estrogen for moisturizing the vagina and maintaining a normal and healthy vaginal pH, Replens contains the chemical compound polycarbophil, which lowers vaginal pH to healthy levels, thus reducing the chance of vaginal infection, says Morris Notelovitz, M.D., in *Menopause and Midlife Health.* Polycarbophil is not found in other vaginal lubricants. Replens can be applied just before intercourse, but the optimum treatment plan is using the gel two or three times a week—regardless of sexual activity—to keep the vagina healthy.

Are the medications we just discussed options for you? It's a subject to discuss in great detail with your doctor—just as you would discuss the use of any new medication. Your medical history, your views about hormone replacement therapy and what you envision as your long-term health goals are all factors that will play a role in your decision, as well as your health care practitioner's knowledge of and opinion about these drugs.

Not to say that you have to take medications. There are nonpharmaceutical approaches for treating menopausal discomforts and helping to prevent health problems later in life. Even if you elect to use a pharmaceutical product, it's worth your while to consider other adjuncts and alternatives to hormone replacement therapy.

Lifestyle Changes As an Alternative to Estrogen

Two lifestyle changes, made in tandem, are variously recommended as an adjunct or an alternative to HRT. These changes entail a new (or renewed) commitment to exercise and to achieving a mineral-rich, nutritionally sound diet.

HRT proponents recommend exercise and a sound diet as adjuncts to HRT because (as we'll see in a moment) these two steps make estrogen work more efficiently. For women who do not wish to take estrogen and other drugs (or cannot take them), a carefully crafted program of exercise and diet can serve as an alternative to HRT, reducing the risk of heart disease and osteoporosis (prevention of which is one of the most persuasive arguments for HRT use) and even helping the body minimize the effects of hot flashes and other vasomotor changes during menopause. Let's see how exercise and diet can improve the health of a woman in menopause and after.

The Role of Exercise

Performed properly and regularly, exercise is one of the best measures you can take to prevent long-term health problems. Exercise reduces the risk of heart disease, and recent evidence suggests that exercise plays a role in preventing breast cancer. Exercise reduces the risk of osteoporosis by halting bone loss—and it does something that HRT does not: *Exercise stimulates the formation of new bone.*

A study of postmenopausal women with low bone density, published in the October 24, 1991, *New England Journal of Medicine,* showed that a regimen of exercise plus calcium supplementation can increase bone mass and slow or prevent bone loss. While the study found that the exercise-calcium regimen was not as effective as an exercise-estrogen regimen, the exercise-estrogen plan caused more side effects.

Beyond this the benefits of exercise are numerous: improved appearance, easier weight control, greater muscle flexibility, better balance, higher energy levels, improved mental well-being, less depression and sounder sleep. Many women find that regular exercise helps curb hot flashes or makes them less severe, possibly by raising the levels of endorphins (natural body chemicals that reduce pain and enhance pleasure) in the brain.

For cardiovascular and osteoporotic protective benefits, exercise should be started at a young age and continued for life. But it's rarely too late to begin an exercise program, as long as you work with your health care practitioner to find the best form of exercise for you.

What type of exercise is best? It should be moderately vigorous—enough to get you to work up a sweat, but not so demanding that it stresses your body or causes injury. As always, check with your doctor before beginning a new exercise program. Here are some of your choices:

Weight-bearing aerobic exercise. Aerobic exercise is a steady activity that gets your heart pumping, conditions the body's muscles and makes you work up a sweat. Weight-bearing aerobic exercises use the weight of your body to put stress on the heart and bones. Brisk walking, jogging, stair climbing, aerobic dancing, skipping rope, bicycling and cross-country skiing, performed for 20 to 30 minutes at a pace brisk enough to accelerate your pulse rate moderately, are ideal options for most women.

Swimming is not considered a weight-bearing exercise, because the water buoyancy takes the stress off bones and joints. Thus, it will have no effect on bone density. But swimming is an excellent low-impact aerobic exercise, thanks to the water buoyancy, which lowers the risk of impact-caused fractures. Swimming is particularly good for older women with painful joints and bones and minor orthopedic problems or for women coming late into an exercise regimen but still hoping to see the heart-healthy and toning effects of exercise.

Regular aerobic exercise strengthens the heart muscle.

Make that aerobic exercise a weight-bearing exercise and you can increase bone density, perhaps as much as 6 percent over two years.

Weight training. If preventing osteoporosis is your goal, then aerobic exercise should be alternated or combined with weight training or muscle-strengthening exercises for your upper body. All the weight-bearing aerobic exercises mentioned earlier work to strengthen the muscles and bones of your lower body, but they don't build bones in your arms and torso. It's important to have healthy, dense bone in your back, for instance, to prevent a curved spine later in life. And strong arm bones will resist fractures in the wrists and lower arms at any age.

Just how does muscle strengthening build thicker, stronger bone? When you stress your muscles with a carefully prepared plan of exercises, the resistance caused by the exercises forces your muscles to enlarge. At the same time that you are stressing your muscles, your muscles are pulling against your bones and stressing them. This stress in turn encourages your bones to grow, absorbing calcium and other minerals from the bloodstream and depositing the calcium and minerals inside the bone to form denser, thicker and stronger bone tissue.

Thus, muscle-strengthening activities result in stronger, calcium-rich bones (as long as your diet includes enough calcium for the bones to absorb, a point we'll discuss later). In contrast, people who are inactive do not stress their bones, and their bones quickly lose calcium, a phenomenon known as bone resorption.

In addition, muscles act as padding. By strengthening your muscles, if you were to fall, your bones would have more protection against fractures.

What exercises are good muscle strengtheners? Your choices include racquetball or tennis, swimming, energetic gardening (lifting and shoveling), modified push-ups, isometric exercises, elastic resistance (using exercise bands), weight lifting with free weights, and weight-training machines. It's not necessary to add a lot of bulk. In fact, it is difficult for the female body to develop the enlarged muscles of the male physique. The goal is to tone muscles and strengthen bones.

Strength training is most effective when done two to three times a week, year-round. Muscles need a 48-hour rest after weight training to recuperate from the gentle stress you have put them through. Year-round training is needed to keep muscles and bones strong. Once you stop, your muscles and bones begin to lose strength.

The key to muscle strengthening is to follow the right exercises and proceed at the proper pace—not too gradually, and definitely not too quickly. Women with painful joints and bones and women with advanced osteoporosis may be unable to launch into a weight-training program. But don't let age alone deter you from "pumping iron." Two researchers at Pennsylvania State University, physiologist William Evans and nutritionist Wayne Campbell, have developed a program for senior citizens consisting of heavy weight lifting and a low-fat, vegetarian diet. In the Penn State program, men and women lift weights three times a week to build muscle, reduce body fat, strengthen bones and achieve better balance and faster walking speed. According to Evans, studies have shown that people in their 90s can triple their strength in less than two months of heavy lifting, enabling them to resume tasks (such as vacuuming, carting laundry and carrying gallon jugs of milk) that they had been forced to discontinue because of loss of strength due to years of inactivity.

Check with your health care practitioner before starting a muscle-strengthening program, and work under the guidance of a trained instructor. Expert advice is crucial when you start a weight-training program.

Balance, or appositive, exercise. New research suggests that slow, concentrated exercises can get the circulation going, improve muscle tone and improve a person's balance. A study of 2,328 elderly people, reported in the May 3, 1995, *Journal of the American Medical Association,* found that elderly people who exercise are less likely to fall. Tai chi, a form of meditative exercise derived from a Chinese martial art, was the most beneficial form of exercise studied, reducing injuries caused by falls by 25 percent. Tai chi is a slow, graceful exercise that emphasizes good balance, making it a healthy option for women even in their 80s and 90s. Yoga is another gentle exercise that can improve balance and increase muscle flexibility in women of all ages.

By combining several types of exercise, you can develop aerobic fitness (benefiting your heart), muscular strength in both your upper and lower body (improving balance) and greater bone density (making debilitating fractures less likely). Exercise is so effective that many doctors advocate a fitness plan for their patients who are on hormone replacement therapy. These doctors note that estrogen works better when a woman is active. And by combining exercise with calcium supplementation, you get additional osteoporotic protection.

Exercise fights osteoporosis only as long as you work out on a regular basis. Once you stop exercising, you begin to lose bone mass. How much is enough? The medical community isn't sure. But the general consensus is that a wise plan, one that maintains bone mass after menopause, entails at least 45 minutes of exercise per session for three to five times a week. Again, develop your personal plan in conjunction with your health care practitioner and a fitness expert.

▌Vaginal Exercises

Urinary incontinence—the tendency to leak urine, especially while laughing, sneezing or coughing—can be a bothersome problem for some women after menopause, when declining levels of estrogen weaken the muscles around the bladder. Then, too, some women report greater difficulty achieving orgasm after menopause.

Estrogen can remedy these problems—but so can exercise. Any exercise that strengthens the back and stomach can tone the muscles that envelop the bladder, urinary tract and vagina. Frequent sexual intercourse (at least once a week) can keep the vaginal lining supple and the muscles surrounding the vagina and urethra (the tube that drains urine from the bladder) firm.

In addition, **Kegel exercises**, also called **pubococcygeus exercises**, strengthen the pubococcygeus muscles, the band of tissue that extends from your pubic bone in the front of your abdomen all the way back to the last four vertebrae in your tailbone. These simple exercises entail squeezing the muscles in the vaginal area for several seconds, then relaxing the muscles, in a squeeze-hold-release-and-repeat pattern. Practice several times a day while sitting, standing or reclining. Kegel exercises improve your ability to retain urine and strengthen the muscles of the vagina, making orgasms possible.

Vitamins, Minerals and the Healthy Diet

The foods that you eat affect the health of your bones and the health of your heart, particularly in the menopausal and postmenopausal years, when many women develop problems with their arteries and bones. A sound nutritional plan, one that takes into account the dietary needs of postmenopausal women, can help keep bones strong and arteries clear.

For women who take HRT, a well-crafted nutritional plan, or diet, is a necessary adjunct to hormone replacement. Without enough calcium, for instance, the bones cannot remain strong, no matter how much estrogen a woman takes.

For some women diet is an alternative to hormone therapy. These women reevaluate and revise their diets in their peri- and postmenopausal years with long-term health in mind. They ensure that they are getting enough vitamins and minerals and are not overloading their systems with too much protein, fat, sugar, caffeine or alcohol. Then they combine this dietary focus with an exercise that improves heart and bone health.

What kind of diet is best? One tailored to your lifestyle and health conditions, of course. Here are a few ideas to consider:

Reduce the amount of protein. Protein inhibits the absorption of calcium and increases the amount of calcium that is excreted from the body in urine. The more protein in your diet, the more calcium your body discharges. According to Robert P. Heaney, M.D., writing in *Calcium and Common Sense,* doubling your protein intake causes 50 percent more calcium to be excreted in your urine. Thus, if you're interested in avoiding osteoporosis, you might reexamine the amount of red meat and other protein you eat. How much is enough? Heaney puts the figure at 44 grams a day for a 120-pound woman, or about half a pound of meat a day (equal to two pieces of fish or skinless poultry, two pork chops or a double hamburger). Other experts put the protein figure lower, estimating that most middle-aged women can get adequate protein from four ounces of lean meat a day. If you wish to eat higher amounts of protein, you need to get additional calcium to counterbalance what the protein causes you to lose.

Avoid "empty" foods. Limit your intake of processed foods (high in fat, sugar and salt), fats, sugar, caffeine and alcohol. Diets that are high in these foods are associated with increased incidence of osteoporosis. Shortly after eating sugar, for instance, your body increases its urinary excretion of calcium. Too much sugar or processed food can change the pH level in your vagina and lead to vaginal infections.

Watch your intake of phosphorus. Around 900 mg of phosphorus a day can help build strong bones. At 1,700 a day or higher, phosphorus can trigger calcium excretion from the bones. Foods containing high amounts of phosphorus are carbonated beverages, red meat and foods processed with phosphorus additives.

Consider a vegetarian diet. Some physicians, including Susan M. Lark, M.D., in *The Menopause Self-Help Book,* recommend a low-fat, high-fiber vegetarian diet, or one close to it, that features cereals, whole grains, beans, vegetables, nuts and seeds. Vegetarian and vegan (no dairy products) diets are associated with a lower risk of osteoporosis, possibly because people on these diets tend to lose less bone mass than people on meat-and-potatoes fare. Studies suggest that vegetarians have the same bone mass as meat eaters in their 20s, 30s and 40s but that people who eat a high volume of meat lose twice as much calcium as vegetarians after age 50, according to sources cited in the *Encyclopedia of Natural Medicine.* The high levels of protein and phosphorus in meat can encourage both bone resorption and long-term bone loss.

Eat foods rich in plant estrogens. The diets of menopausal women should include foods that are high in **phytoestrogens**, chemicals that the body converts into estrogen. Phytoestrogens (sometimes called **plant estrogens**, although they are not actually estrogen itself) seem to have the ability to diminish menopausal discomforts. Although phytoestrogens contain less than 1/400th of the amount of estrogen in a hormone supplement, the cumulative effect of a diet of weakly estrogenic foods may offer some protection against menopausal discomforts and possibly against osteoporosis and heart disease.

Foods high in phytoestrogens include soy products (soybeans, tofu, miso), papaya and yams. Lesser amounts can be found in apples, brown rice, carrots, green beans, peas, potatoes, red beans, sesame seeds, whole wheat and rye, according to an article in *Alternative Medicine: The Definitive Guide.*

Colorful and aromatic compounds called **flavonoids** (also known as bioflavonoids) are found in fruit. Flavonoids also are weak plant estrogens instrumental in stabilizing collagen, the major protein structure in bone. Flavonoids can be found in blackberries, blueberries, cherries, raspberries, citrus rinds and other deeply colored fruits.

(continued on page 178)

▌ Plant Estrogens—Friend or Foe?

Many herbs that have been used for centuries to relieve hot flashes and other menopause-related discomforts happen to be sources of plant estrogen. Some herbs such as ginseng are relatively potent phytoestrogens; others such as red clover are relatively weak. If you use phyto-estrogenic herbs and eat phytoestrogenic foods, are you actually taking a form of estrogen replacement therapy?

Some doctors say yes, arguing that natural estrogen is still estrogen and can have the same positive—and negative—effects as estrogen pills, patches or creams. What makes phytoestrogens potentially dangerous, these doctor argue, is that you can't tell how much estrogen you're getting. When you eat plant estrogens or take phytoestrogenic herbs, doses can't be tightly controlled the way they can be with a pharmaceutical preparation.

Alternative practitioners point out, however, that phytoestrogens are not estrogens per se, although they are chemicals that the body can convert into estrogen. In addition, phytoestrogens are considerably weaker than estrogen as taken in HRT; plant estrogens offer only 1/400th of a dose of pharmaceutically prepared estrogen. Moreover, Michael Murray, N.D., and Joseph Pizzorno, N.D., writing in the *Encyclopedia of Natural Medicine*, point out that phytoestrogens tend to balance estrogen levels in the body. If estrogen levels are low, they say, phytoestrogens will cause an increase in estrogen effect. If estrogen levels are high, phytoestrogens will compete with estrogen to bind onto estrogen receptor sites in the body, thus decreasing estrogen effects.

▼

If you're considering taking plant estrogens to relieve menopausal discomforts, be sure to discuss it with your doctor—just as you would discuss any health strategy. It's especially important to talk with your doctor if you have been advised not to take estrogen (perhaps you have a history of estrogen-dependent cancer) or if you have any other contraindication for hormone replacement therapy. (See Chapter 3.)

You may seek to get all your vitamins and minerals from the foods you eat, but this is sometimes difficult (particularly in the case of calcium). Some women use vitamin and mineral supplements, but this should be done carefully and in conjunction with your health care practitioner. (Some vitamins, such as vitamins A, B_6 and D, can be harmful when taken in extra-large doses.) Whether you get your vitamins and minerals from your diet, from supplements or a combination of the two, the experts agree that your diet should include enough of the following:

• **Calcium.** Representing about 40 percent of all the minerals found in your bones, calcium is responsible for bone strength. Your body also uses calcium to maintain brain function, aid in muscle contraction and assist in clotting blood. If you don't take in enough calcium in your daily diet, your body begins to siphon from the bones the calcium it needs to do its other jobs.

Nutritionists today say that most American women only get from 500 to 700 mg of calcium a day—not nearly enough to prevent bone resorption. To prevent bone resorption, premenopausal women need at least 1,000 mg of calcium a day. After menopause, women need at least 1,000 mg of calcium a day if they take estrogen and at least 1,500 mg if they do not (*Current Obstetric and Gynecologic Diagnosis and Treatment*).

Drinking three or four cups of milk (at 350 mg of calcium a cup) a day is one way to get your calcium. Eating calcium-rich foods is another. These foods include a cup of cooked collard greens, eight canned sardines, a cup of calcium-fortified orange juice and a cup of yogurt (regular or low fat), all of which contain at least 300 mg of calcium. Lesser amounts of calcium are found in the average servings of such foods as tahini, canned salmon (with bones) and cooked broccoli. Taking calcium supplements is the third way to ensure your bones have the needed calcium. Since you may not like or be able to tolerate milk, and it is hard to get enough calcium from other food sources, you may well be among the many American women who need to take daily calcium supplements.

Eating plenty of calcium-rich foods or taking calcium supplements will not replenish lost bone mass, but it can slow bone loss. For best results, however, you need to take adequate amounts of vitamins D, C, K and the mineral magnesium to ensure calcium absorption. Exercise enhances absorption, as does estrogen. In contrast, inactivity, illness, some medications, caffeine, some foods and cigarette smoking can impede (but not necessarily stop) calcium absorption, meaning you may need to take even more calcium. Check with your doctor or a nutritionist for more details.

• **Vitamin D.** The right amount of vitamin D helps your body absorb calcium. Sheldon H. Cherry, M.D., and

Carolyn C. Runowicz, M.D., recommend approximately 400 international units per day (*The Menopause Book*). Too much vitamin D (over 1,000 units per day) can cause bone loss. Young women and women active in the outdoors usually get enough vitamin D. As people age, the amount of vitamin D circulating in their blood decreases by nearly 50 percent, the side effect of an age-related deficiency of an enzyme produced by the kidneys. This may account for why elderly women and women with osteoporosis often have a vitamin D deficiency.

You can get vitamin D from being in the sun or from your diet. Sunlight promotes the manufacture of natural vitamin D in your body. Somewhere between 15 and 60 minutes of sunlight on your skin is needed to get your daily dose. The exact amount of time is impossible to gauge, but in general women in northern climates require more exposure than women in southern climes, simply because the sun's rays weaken as you move north of the equator. In winter when the sun's rays are at their lowest and when cold temperatures keep people indoors, it may be difficult to get enough sunlight to generate your needed vitamin D. In that case you can turn to foods rich in this vitamin.

Dietary sources of vitamin D include fatty fish (halibut, mackerel, salmon), vitamin-D-enriched milk, liver, butter and egg yolks (the latter three being, unfortunately, the sorts of cholesterol-laden food that women should try to avoid). If you can't get enough vitamin D from exposure to the sun or from food sources, you may need a vitamin supplement. Ask your doctor for a recommendation.

In a nutshell, calcium and vitamin D are essential partners in preventing fractures. Together they are sometimes seen as an alternative therapy to estrogen.

• **Magnesium.** As mentioned earlier, calcium and vitamin D work in concert with magnesium. Found in bone tissue, magnesium plays a role in bone formation and in muscle contraction. The proper amount of magnesium helps the body use vitamin D to build strong bones. Too little or too much magnesium impairs bone calcification and growth.

The recommended balance of magnesium and calcium is two parts of calcium to one part magnesium. If you take 1,500 mg of calcium, you need about 750 mg of magnesium. This ratio hold true for women in the pre-, peri- and postmenopausal years. Many calcium supplements come with magnesium added in these correct amounts.

You can get magnesium from certain foods, including dark green vegetables, shellfish, legumes, cereals and nuts. Or you can take a mineral supplement; ask your health care practitioner to recommend one.

• **Vitamin K.** This vitamin helps keep calcium in place within the bone. Without vitamin K, bones can't mineralize (form). This vitamin is abundant in leafy green vegetables. For those who don't eat their greens, fat-soluble chlorophyll capsules (available at natural foods stores) are another source of vitamin K. You don't need a lot of vitamin K to keep your bones healthy, so supplements are rarely necessary.

• **Vitamin E.** Not just a necessary nutrient, vitamin E is also used as an alternative therapy by **herbalists** (persons skilled in the art of herbal medicine who can compound herbal mixtures made from plants) and naturopathic physicians to treat hot flashes. It is also an adjunct therapy prescribed by mainstream medical practitioners.

Some experts believe that vitamin E can relieve hot flashes and other vasomotor symptoms. Taken in amounts of 400 international units several times a day, for a total of 800 to 1,600 units a day, vitamin E can produce for some women a remarkable decrease in the severity and frequency of symptoms.

Vitamin E vaginal creams are also available to combat the problems of atrophic vaginitis (the shrinkage of vaginal tissues after menopause that can make sexual intercourse uncomfortable). These creams are often more effective than vaginal lubricants and perhaps as effective as the vaginal moisturizer Replens.

Vitamin E is found in such foods as whole grains and cereals, nuts, and wheat germ and safflower oils. It's nearly impossible to get 800 to 1,600 international units of vitamin E from dietary sources; most women also need to take supplements.

• **B vitamins and vitamin C.** Low levels of vitamins B and C are common in elderly people, and some scientists believe this may play a role in the development of osteoporosis. Additionally some women report that these vitamins can take the edge off menopausal discomforts, although there is no medical consensus on whether this really works. A practitioner who is a believer may recommend a vitamin B-complex tablet and suggest the ideal dosage (often between 500 and 1,000 mg a day) of vitamin C.

The Alternative Therapies

A combination of exercise, diet, and vitamin and mineral supplementation can be seen as an alternative or adjunct to hormone replacement therapy. Many other alternative therapies are available to help women who take care of their health before, during and after the menopausal years. The problem with these therapies—bear in mind that some women do not consider this a problem—is that few have been tested in clinical studies. Thus, there is little scientific evidence for evaluating how effective (or ineffective) these therapies may be.

That said, it's important to note that some alternative practitioners are also M.D.'s or D.O.'s—meaning that they combine traditional allopathic or osteopathic (that is, scientific) medicine with elements of alternative therapies. A woman who wants to explore an alternative treatment for menopause-related conditions, but who is loath to abandon the mainstream medical system, may wish to start with a consultation with just such a doctor.

Let's look at some of the available therapies:

Homeopathy

Homeopathic medicine treats illnesses by using safe and very tiny doses of natural medicines, extracted from plants, animal material or natural chemicals, to stimulate a person's own healing powers while avoiding harmful side effects. Most homeopathic physicians in practice today are medical doctors or doctors of osteopathy who have additional training in homeopathic principles. There are more than 500 M.D.'s and D.O.'s who include homeopathic principles in their practice of medicine, according to the National Center for Homeopathy. Other health care practitioners, such as nurse practitioners, nurse-midwives, physician assistants, licensed acupuncturists and naturopathic physicians, may be allowed to use homeopathy within the scope of their licenses, depending on the laws of the state in which they reside. To determine if a homeopathic physician you are considering is also an M.D. or D.O., contact the National Center for Homeopathy. (See the Resources section at the back of this book.)

According to Andrew Lockie, M.D., and Nicola Geddes, M.D., in *The Women's Guide to Homeopathy,* "The homeopathic view of menopausal problems is that they represent imbalances which have been present for a long time; treatment is therefore constitutional." The authors advise preparing for menopause by reevaluating your diet and exercise plan and developing a positive attitude toward menopause.

Homeopathic physicians have over 3,000 remedies in their lexicon, each designed to treat very specific complaints. And because each remedy or dose must be individualized to each woman, homeopaths are loath to recommend general therapies for menopausal women. Lockie and Geddes note that remedies exist that can be used as a homeopathic HRT, but they believe these should be used only under the guidance of an experienced homeopath.

Homeopathic medicine doesn't exclude the use of vitamins, nutritional supplements or allopathic (scientific) medications prescribed by physicians, says Rebecca Elmaleth, M.D., interviewed in *Without Estrogen: Natural Remedies for Menopause and Beyond.* Homeopathy "balances and stabilizes a body going through natural changes," she says. Indeed, allopathic treatments may sometimes be necessary. For instance, Elmaleth acknowledges that homeopathy may not be the best form of treatment for osteoporosis, "because there are no symptoms until the condition is well established." She adds: "Homeopathy would never make the condition worse, but we can't say if what we do arrests the condition or prevents it."

Naturopathy

Naturopathy is a healing art that emphasizes the body's natural healing forces. A doctor of naturopathic medicine

(N.D.) uses your medical history to make a diagnosis, supplemented by laboratory tests and other diagnostic techniques such as x-rays, scans and physicals. Once a diagnosis is made, the naturopath sets about restoring health by taking the whole person into account and not just the symptoms. Naturopaths consider diet and nutrition to be essential to good health, and they advise patients on the types of food to eat as well as those to avoid.

An M.D. or D.O. can become a naturopath by getting additional training in naturopathic principles. Further, eight states license non-M.D. and non-D.O. naturopathic physicians to diagnose and treat illness.

To prevent osteoporosis, or stop its progression, naturopaths devise a regimen of exercise, diet, vitamin and mineral supplementation and botanical herbs. Michael Murray, N.D., and Joseph Pizzorno, N.D., writing in the *Encyclopedia of Natural Medicine,* propose a plan of walking 45 to 60 minutes three to five times a week; a high-fiber, low-fat, low-meat diet, with restricted intake of refined carbohydrates, alcohol and carbonated beverages; supplements of calcium, magnesium, vitamin B_{12}, folic acid and vitamin K, among others; and use of botanical medicines such as dried roots, tinctures or extracts to treat menopausal symptoms.

To treat atrophic vaginitis, Murray and Pizzorno recommend a low-fat, nutrient-rich diet with no refined foods or simple carbohydrates such as sugar; supplements of B-complex vitamins and vitamin E; topical vitamin E cream; and use of phytoestrogenic foods and herbs.

Herbs and botanical medicines are a cornerstone of naturopathic medicine as well as other alternative therapies such as herbal medicine (a healing art that uses plants to prevent and cure illnesses) and Chinese medicine (which also includes massage and **acupuncture**). Before allopathic (scientific) medicine gained the upper hand early in this century, both herbology and allopathy existed side by side. Today, however, the scientific faction views herbology as folk medicine or just plain quackery.

Which herbs are thought to be most effective in addressing menopausal discomforts? Here are several:

• **Dong quai.** This herb has been prepared for hundreds of years by Chinese doctors to alleviate hot flashes and is one of the most common herbs for treating "female complaints" in this country as well as abroad. Dong quai is a phytoestrogen (a plant containing chemicals that the body converts into estrogen).

• **Ginseng.** Another plant estrogen, ginseng is used by Chinese herbalists to treat menopausal discomforts, stimulate the immune system, normalize blood pressure and reduce cholesterol levels, writes Dee Ito in *Without Estrogen: Natural Remedies for Menopause and Beyond.* Ito notes that ginseng has an anticlotting effect that may reduce the risk of heart attack, has a protective effect on the liver and is rich in vitamins A, E and B_{12} and calcium. Three types of ginseng are available in the United States, Ito writes— Chinese, Korean and Siberian. As each comes in different strengths, you'll need the assistance of an herbalist to determine the best type for you. As for side effects, ginseng has been known to disrupt sleep when taken late at night.

• **Black cohosh.** The root of this phytoestrogenic herb is used to relieve hot flashes and vaginal dryness. Black cohosh is an ingredient in three drugs prescribed in Germany for treating menopausal symptoms, writes Michael Castleman in *The Healing Herbs: The Ultimate Guide to the Curative Power of Nature's Medicines.* Here in the United

States, Castleman says, the Food and Drug Administration states that black cohosh has no therapeutic value and warns of overdoses that could cause dizziness, nausea, vomiting, headache and a depressed heart rate.

• **False unicorn.** The root of this phytoestrogenic herb can lift depression, soothe headaches and stimulate the reproductive organs, says Ito in *Without Estrogen.*

• **Fennel.** This plant estrogen has a long historical use in treating menopausal complaints, according to the *Encyclopedia of Natural Medicine.* As for side effects, Castleman in *The Healing Herbs* points to a study suggesting that fennel can disturb the liver, making medicinal doses of this herb inappropriate for anyone with a history of liver disease.

• **Licorice.** This root is a phytoestrogen that can be used to treat hot flashes. Ito says that it is often used together with sarsaparilla root, as the sarsaparilla contains progesterone and helps balance the effects of licorice. Increased energy levels and reduced stress are benefits that can be derived from licorice, but it can also raise blood pressure.

• **Anise.** Because anise seed contains phytoestrogens it may help relieve menopausal discomforts, Castleman says. He notes that the FDA considers anise to be safe, but he says that high doses of this herb—several teaspoons—can cause nausea and vomiting.

• **Red clover.** This plant can act like estrogen when taken in large quantities. The FDA considers red clover to be safe, Castleman writes, though this plant can sometimes cause mild stomach upset or diarrhea.

• **Motherwort.** An aid in relieving palpitations that accompany hot flashes, motherwort is also a good herb to

(continued on page 189)

■ The Right Practitioner: Questions to Ask

Whether you choose to be treated in the mainstream medical system or in an alternative setting, always work in concert with a knowledgeable physician or practitioner. Contact the appropriate state licensing board (if there is one) to find out what credentials are needed to get a license. Verify that the practitioner is licensed. Call the practitioner's professional organization for more details on evaluating practitioners. (Some of these organizations are listed in the Resources section of this book.)

Whomever you choose to help you in managing your health in your menopausal and postmenopausal years, be sure you ask the practitioner at least the following questions:

- What is your training in women's health?

- Are you licensed to practice in this state, and if so what state board gave you the license?

- How many menopausal patients do you have?

- Are they using the same therapy you are recommending to me?

- How long do they stay on it?

- What kinds of problems do you see among them?

- Should I be seeing another doctor who specializes in this area?

- What health risks does this treatment pose? What benefits?

- In light of my personal medical history, will this treatment increase those risks?

▼

> • What will this treatment do for me? In what way?
>
> • What are the common side effects of the regimen you are recommending?
>
> • Should I be monitored for possible problems? What form will this monitoring take?
>
> • If I decide to try this therapy, when should I start?
>
> • How much time do I have to make this decision?
>
> Add more questions to this list as you think of them.

help women wean themselves off hormone replacement therapy, says Diane Stein in *The Natural Remedy Book for Women*. She discusses how motherwort can ease the transition and keep your body from slipping into a state of hormonal imbalance.

• **Chamomile.** This herb, often served as a tea, is a relaxant, according to *The Dictionary of Modern Herbalism*. As is true of lemon verbena, woodruff, hawthorn, hops and passionflower, chamomile as an herb may help menopausal women who are particularly anxious, agitated, restless and sleepless, says Andrew Lockie, M.D., and Nicola Geddes, M.D., in *The Women's Guide to Homeopathy*.

There are many other herbs that can be used during and after menopause, including alfalfa for relieving water retention and bloatedness, juniper berries and buchu leaves for urinary incontinence and wild Mexican yam (which contains a natural progesterone) for relief of anxiety.

Many alternative doctors (including homeopathic, naturopathic and herbal) recommend herbs in combinations. Andrew Weil offers an herbal formula for hot flashes in his book *Natural Health, Natural Medicine.* Susan Lark, M.D., offers three herbal formulas in *The Menopause Self-Help Book.* (Turn to the Resources and Bibliography sections for more information on these and other resources.) Rather than diagnosing yourself, however, most alternative practitioners recommend that you get a specific, personalized botanical formula based on a diagnosis of your particular menopausal symptoms, medical history and overall health. While most herbs are safe in moderation, some can cause unexpected reactions (allergic or toxic) if taken in too large or too frequent a dose.

Acupuncture and Acupressure

Acupuncture is an ancient Chinese healing art in which very thin needles are inserted under the skin, at specific acupuncture sites on the body, to treat illness and restore good health. Chinese medicine (which also includes massage and herbal medicine) teaches that in order to remain healthy, yin and yang (negative and positive forces) must be perfectly balanced and that it is necessary to have a flow of a life force, known as chi, throughout the body. The chi flows along paths known as meridians (sets of invisible lines) and covers the body in set patterns. While meridians are not identical to the nervous system or circulatory system, they are thought to resemble them. When illness occurs, the acupuncturist examines the meridians and carefully selects acupuncture sites. It is at these sites that acupuncture is given.

Some women try acupuncture and find that it helps re-

lieve the severity and frequency of flashes and other vasomotor symptoms.

Acupressure, another form of Chinese medicine, is
therapy in which the fingers rather than needles are used to
apply pressure along the meridians. By stimulating the acupressure points along the meridians, life forces are per-
mitted to flow to various parts of the body.

According to *Acupressure for Everybody* by Cathryn
Bauer, Asian medical practitioners treat hot flashes by
pressing "cooling points" on the foot and hand to balance
body temperature.

Biofeedback

This is a psychological therapy that uses the conscious
mind to control involuntary body functions such as respiration, heartbeat and body temperature. After being trained
in biofeedback, some menopausal women are able to reduce the frequency and severity of their hot flashes.
Biofeedback can also be used as a relaxation technique.

Biofeedback can be learned by anyone, but the techniques used to train someone in the use of biofeedback
have become very sophisticated. Often these techniques are
learned at a medical center or a clinic where certified instructors specialize in teaching people this therapy. Using
high-tech equipment, the practitioner can monitor brain
impulses and make them audible to the woman who is
using biofeedback. By monitoring this electrical activity and
listening to a series of beeps, the woman learns how to control the situation. (See the Resources section for information on biofeedback instructors.)

As we mentioned, some women use biofeedback to

control hot flashes and body temperature. Biofeedback has also been employed for stress headaches, migraine headaches and back pain.

There are other healing arts—including Chinese medicine, Ayurvedic medicine (a holistic medicine originating in India) and Bach flower remedies (a form of herbal medicine)—that may have approaches to help you cope with menopause and menopausal discomforts. A thorough discussion of these is outside the scope of this book, but you can turn to the Resources section for sources of further information on these therapies.

Self-Help

There are hundreds of self-help strategies that women use as alternatives or adjuncts to estrogen for coping with menopausal discomforts. They include tips for reducing hot flashes, such as keeping a food diary to determine if certain foods or beverages trigger flashes; keeping your home and workplace cool (65 to 68 degrees); and wearing layers of thin clothing so you can shed items during hot flashes.

To prevent vaginal infections, you can douche with a plain lactobacillus acidophilus yogurt. To prevent urinary tract infections, you can drink eight glasses of water a day, drink cranberry juice and wear cotton-crotch underwear.

Since the focus of this book is on hormones, we aren't able to give you a complete guide (if one could ever be compiled!) to self-help strategies. For a list of many excellent books that discuss these strategies in detail, see the Bibliography section at the back of this book.

What's Next?

As you've seen in this chapter, you have many options to HRT during your menopausal and postmenopausal years. Most of these entail making a commitment to a healthy lifestyle—changing the way you exercise and eat. If you are willing to take more responsibility for your health, you may be able to circumvent HRT by making substantial and beneficial life changes. Many of these changes have no negative side effects.

Deciding whether to take hormone replacement therapy or to try an alternative approach can be a difficult process, even with all the information you've been given so far. The next chapter will summarize the major arguments for and against hormone replacement and help you pull all the pieces together so you can make an informed decision.

CHAPTER VII

Weighing Your Choices

W hen you opened this book you entered the debate over one of the most controversial issues of female health care. There are persuasive arguments for and against hormone replacement therapy—with studies to back up each view. And if there's anything we have learned so far, it's that there is little agreement between experts.

So where does this leave you? Admittedly some women are so overwhelmed by the contradictions that they elect to do nothing. Other women pick a side and go for it, knowing that it's okay to change their minds later as findings from new research come to light.

You can, in fact, try HRT, stop it, then resume it, just as you can try an alternative therapy and then switch to HRT later in life. Ideally the decision should be made in concert with your health care practitioner.

To help you weigh all sides, let's summarize some of the key arguments for and against hormone replacement therapy's short-term and long-term uses.

The Points for Prevention

Among the most persuasive arguments for the use of HRT as a preventive:

HRT quickly relieves vasomotor discomforts. It is universally agreed that HRT has a long history of controlling or alleviating physical discomforts caused by the estrogen deficiency that begins at menopause. These include hot flashes, drenching sweats, the sensation of crawling skin and other vasomotor symptoms. Some research suggests that HRT can improve mental well-being and combat depression in menopausal and postmenopausal women, while many experts contest these findings.

HRT combats atrophy or shrinking of the tissues. Without estrogen, tissues in the vagina, bladder, muscles, breasts and skin shrink and begin to lose their resilience. In many women this situation gradually leads to a dry and easily irritated vagina (atrophic vaginitis), more frequent vaginal and urinary infections, decreasing muscle strength, sagging breasts and drier and looser skin. By replenishing the body with estrogen through HRT, vaginal and urinary infections are less likely to occur and muscle tone is easier to maintain; and although estrogen doesn't prevent aging and wrinkling, it helps maintain a cushion of oil-producing collagen under the skin, making it seem more flexible and younger.

HRT protects against heart disease. Heart disease is the number one cause of death in women over age 50. Based on studies so far, it appears that HRT may lower the risk of heart disease by 50 percent. In light of this statistic, HRT advocates argue that for most women hormone replacement provides heart benefits that far outweigh the known risks. Women with a family history of heart attack or stroke or who currently have a heart condition may elect to use HRT, hoping that its protective benefits are indeed as positive as these new studies predict.

HRT protects against osteoporosis. HRT cannot repair damaged bone, but it has clearly been shown to arrest the progression of osteoporosis. For women who are at high risk of osteoporosis (Caucasian or Asian race, small body frame, parent with low bone mass and other risk factors), HRT can be a godsend. The most recent evidence suggests that long-term use of HRT can reduce the incidence of osteoporotic hip and wrist fractures by 60 percent.

HRT improves quality of life and extends life expectancy. By alleviating menopausal symptoms and protecting against bone loss, bone fractures and heart disease, HRT improves the quality of a woman's life and even can extend her life expectancy, HRT advocates argue. There is some evidence for this assumption: In the February 1994 *American Journal of Obstetrics and Gynecology,* a French study of 499 postmenopausal women compared the responses of those using the transdermal estrogen patch with those who were given the drug verapipride (a European drug that treats hot flashes). Both groups of women completed questionnaires before and after treatment. After six months of therapy, the women on HRT reported an overall improved quality of life and general feelings of well-being, with marked improvements in the quality of sleep and sex life, and less anxiety.

And there is some substance to the claim that HRT extends life expectancy. An epidemiologic study reported in the March 1993 *Journal of Family Practice* estimated that among women at low risk of developing cardiovascular disease, hormone therapy may extend life .3 year; among women at high risk, HRT may extend life 2.3 years.

If you have debilitating menopausal symptoms or frequent vaginal or urinary infections, or if you are at high risk of osteoporosis or heart disease, these arguments make sense and may make up your mind. If you don't know your personal risks, or if you are at low, average or moderate risk, you may be on the fence about HRT—attracted by the potential benefits, but concerned about the potential risks. Let's review those risks now.

HRT Concerns From B to W

HRT offers real benefits. But for most women these benefits are not achieved without some adverse effects. They can be short-term side effects (such as withdrawal bleeding) or long-term hazards (such as a greater risk of breast cancer). In addition, there are situations in which HRT should not be used (absolute contraindications) and situations in which HRT should be used with care (relative contraindications). We call all of these "HRT concerns."

You've met these concerns earlier in this book. Which ones apply to you? The answer will depend upon your personal medical history as well as your overall health. For the purpose of review, we bring them to your attention once again, this time arranged in alphabetical order:

• *Blood clotting (thrombosis)* is an absolute contraindication to HRT when the clots have occurred in the recent past. The concern is that estrogen may decrease the anti-clotting factors of the blood, so that women on HRT who tend to develop clots might experience thrombophlebitis (a blood clot and an inflammation in a vein, such as in a leg) or thromboembolism (a clot that breaks away and travels to the lungs, heart or brain, where it blocks a blood vessel), leading to heart attack or stroke. In contrast, varicose veins and hemorrhoids are not considered contraindications to HRT.

What if you had thrombophlebitis in the past, but have had no problems in recent years—could you use HRT? Not if hormone use triggered the condition in the past. If previous thrombophlebitis was not hormone related, the answer is less clear. Some practitioners believe that the transdermal patch or a vaginal estrogen cream are two options for women susceptible to clotting, as long as those women are given blood tests to be sure their anticlotting factors are normal. Research published in the December 1993 *American Journal of Obstetrics and Gynecology* confirmed the hypothesis that current doses of HRT do not appear to cause blood clots.

• *Breast cancer* is an absolute contraindication for HRT and the most controversial aspect of hormone replacement. Over 30 studies have investigated the possibility of a connection between HRT and breast cancer, and researchers still dispute the findings. The latest support for a link between long-term HRT use and breast cancer comes from a Harvard Medical School study published in the June 15, 1995, *New England Journal of Medicine,* which found that postmenopausal women on estrogen for more than five years had a 32 percent higher risk of developing breast cancer than those who had never taken hormones. The highest risk—71 percent—appeared in women ages 60 to 64. The study's authors write, "The substantial increase in the risk of breast cancer among older women who take hormones suggests that the trade-offs between risks and benefits should be carefully assessed."

• *Breast tenderness and swelling,* called mastalgia in medical lingo, is a side effect of estrogen. Mastalgia may disappear a few months after starting HRT, or it can remain. Some women are so uncomfortable that their medical practitioners prescribe testosterone (a male hormone also found in the female body), which relieves painful breasts. Testosterone has side effects of its own, including decreasing HDL cholesterol (the good cholesterol) levels and, occasionally, encouraging the growth of facial hair.

• *Cholesterol* levels in the blood are affected by estrogen. In particular, estrogen appears to reduce levels of harmful cholesterol (LDL cholesterol) and increase levels of beneficial cholesterol (HDL cholesterol) in the blood, thus giving a measure of protection against heart disease among women who are susceptible to the disease.

Research published in the January 18, 1995, *Journal of the American Medical Association* suggests that some of this protection is lost when progestin is taken with estrogen—particularly medroxyprogesterone acetate, the progestin most frequently prescribed in the United States. It appears that progestin decreases HDL cholesterol, muting—but not canceling out—the heart-healthy benefit of estrogen.

• *Chronic headaches* are a side effect of the progestin component in estrogen-progestin HRT. They can develop into migraine headaches. For some women the chronic headaches are severe enough to cause them to quit HRT or for their practitioners to recommend taking small doses of testosterone, which can prevent the headaches.

• *Depression* is a side effect of progestin. If it develops it may be relieved by lowering the progestin dose or by discontinuing the progestin altogether.

• *Diabetes* is a relative contraindication to HRT, meaning that HRT can sometimes make this condition worse by disturbing blood sugar levels. In a diabetic postmenopausal woman who has her diabetes under control, HRT may not pose a problem. But for someone who has diabetes and does not know it or for someone with severe complications of diabetes, estrogen may wreak havoc with blood sugar levels.

• *Endometrial cancer* is an absolute contraindication for HRT use. Estrogen encourages endometrial cancer's growth. Estrogen can even cause endometrial cancer by encouraging the proliferation of cells in the endometrium (lining of the uterus). One form of HRT, known as unopposed estrogen therapy, increases the risk of endometrial cancer two- to fifteenfold in women who still have a uterus.

• *Endometriosis* is a relative contraindication to HRT. It occurs when cells from the endometrium migrate outside the uterus, where they grow on other organs within the abdomen when stimulated by estrogen and progestin. Endometriosis may disappear after menopause when estrogen and progesterone levels fall. For that reason health care practitioners often withhold HRT from women with endometriosis for three to 12 months after menopause. The idea is to give the migrated endometrial cells time to wither and die, so that the woman can then use estrogen without stimulating the migrated cells.

• *Fibroids* are relative contraindications. These noncancerous uterine tumors, found in half of women over age 50, usually shrink on their own after menopause when estrogen levels fall. Because estrogen stimulates fibroid growth, some women with large fibroids choose not to take HRT. Other women wait two or three years before starting HRT to give their fibroids time to wither and shrink. Still other women are willing to try low-dose hormone replacement, particularly if their fibroids are small and not troublesome. If while on HRT you develop fibroids that cause heavy bleeding, abdominal pain or uncomfortable pressure on your bladder or bowel, then you'll have to discontinue HRT. You probably won't be able to resume it.

• *Gallbladder disease* is a relative contraindication to HRT. Research suggests that women on estrogen are two and one-half times more likely to develop gallstones. Estrogen encourages increased amounts of cholesterol to collect in the bile manufactured by the liver, eventually forming cholesterol-based gallstones.

Scientists today think that estrogen in the form of pills and tablets is more likely to lead to gallstones in women susceptible to gallbladder problems than estrogen in the form of transdermal patches. If you have a history of gallbladder disease or gallstones and you choose to try HRT, you may want to use transdermal patches and be sure your doctor monitors the effects of therapy on your body.

• *High blood pressure* is a relative contraindication. Estrogen encourages the kidneys to produce angiotensin, a chemical that causes blood vessels to narrow. In turn blood pressure can increase, a situation that doctors call estrogen-associated hypertension. This problem is more common with oral contraceptives than with the estrogens used in HRT, but women with hypertension need to be aware that estrogen could affect their blood pressure readings.

• *Liver disease or chronic impaired liver function* is an absolute contraindication to hormone therapy. When estrogen is taken orally, it is processed by the liver before it goes into the bloodstream. An impaired or diseased liver may not convert estrogen properly; in turn the estrogen may become a toxin in the body. A past history of liver disease is not necessarily an absolute contraindication. Some doctors believe that vaginal estrogen creams and transdermal patches are safe for women who do not have active liver disease, because the estrogen in the creams and patches is *not* taken orally and thus the estrogen bypasses the liver.

• *Migraines* can (but don't always) worsen under HRT. Thus, migraines headaches are considered a relative contraindication. Reducing the amount of estrogen you take may solve the problem. But if migraines persist, the benefits of HRT may not be worth the head pain.

• *Nausea and vomiting* are occasional side effects of the progestin component of combination therapy.

• *Seizure disorders* are a relative contraindication. If a woman already experiences seizures, they may become more frequent when she takes HRT, possibly due to the way that estrogen encourages water retention in the brain.

• *Withdrawal bleeding* is a side effect of HRT in a cyclic or sequential combination regimen—that is, estrogen with progestin on certain days of the month. It occurs after progestin is discontinued (withdrawn) each month and mimics a menstrual period. Eighty to 90 percent of women who begin taking cyclic estrogen plus progestin regain their periods. These periods generally last from two to five days and gradually lighten over time. Although the periods eventually disappear, withdrawal bleeding is unpopular. It is listed as the number one reason that women stop HRT therapy.

Women aren't the only ones concerned about side effects. Doctors, too, debate the benefits and the risks of hormone replacement, particularly long-term HRT.

The Arguments for Short-Term Use or Alternative Therapies

Few physicians dispute the claims that HRT can make the menopausal years easier by relieving discomforts; few dispute findings that the bones and heart appear to benefit from estrogen. Strictly looking at statistics, most mainstream medical practitioners believe that the benefits of hormone replacement far outweigh the risks. But statistics apply to large groups of people; they don't predict what will happen to the individual woman.

Thus, while some practitioners suggest that HRT is suitable for every woman (with very few exceptions), other practitioners argue a conservative approach, prescribing HRT only for those at-risk women who have a clear need for the assistance estrogen offers and for whom alternatives to HRT are not appropriate or successful. These conservative practitioners want to wait until the evidence about HRT risks is clear; they don't want to unnecessarily expose women to unknown or unclear risks that may one day outweigh the benefits of HRT. So they call for greater emphasis on known preventive strategies such as improved diet and regular exercise. Here are highlights of their arguments:

There is rising concern over long-term health hazards associated with HRT. These long-term hazards include breast cancer, which we discussed earlier. Many alternative therapies offer benefits without these risks.

Lower risk factors may not necessarily prevent illness or lengthen life. The January 18, 1995, issue of the *Journal of the American Medical Association* published findings showing that some forms of hormone replacement therapy can indeed reduce key cardiovascular risk factors in women over age 50. But even the physicians who participated in the study acknowledge that it hasn't been shown that the improvements in cardiovascular risk factors linked to HRT will actually translate into fewer heart attacks and strokes. The answer may not be known until the Women's Health Initiative, devised by the National Institutes of Health to evaluate HRT and other female health issues, releases data sometime in the year 2005.

Past studies of HRT did not eliminate bias. There has been concern that studies of HRT and its effects on health may not accurately reflect reality because the type of woman who has traditionally used HRT does not reflect the general American population. An abstract published in the February 1993 *Circulation* joins the ranks of several articles reporting that women taking hormone therapy tend to be healthier and wealthier than women not taking HRT. If this is true, it could be that the benefits of HRT have been inflated because sicker women were not given these drugs.

In the December 1993 *Obstetrics and Gynecology,* two Finnish authors examined prescribing advice given from 1945 to 1990 to U.S. physicians through the *Physicians' Desk Reference* (the medical industry bible of prescription drug uses, side effects and contraindications), five medical textbooks and other sources. The authors found that over the years since 1970, prescribing advice has recommended that physicians not give estrogens to women in poor general health. As authors Elina Hemminki, M.D., and Sinikka Sihvo, M.P.H., explain, "If the advice observed reflects the prescribing practices of physicians, then surveys on the health impact of estrogen therapy may have underestimated the risk of breast cancer and overestimated the prevention of fractures."

In other words, doctors for years may have been giving HRT to women who were healthy and not giving HRT to women in poor health. Thus, the good results that HRT appeared to achieve were in part due to the already good health of the women taking hormones. If less healthy women had been taking HRT too, this argument goes, then the reports of HRT's benefits might have been less glowing.

Hormones are being prescribed to women who are not at risk or who are at low risk. Critics of the marketing of menopause as disease raise serious questions about the wisdom of putting *most* women on hormone therapy when only some women are at risk.

A call for reconsideration of HRT use was written by Lynn Rosenberg, Sc.D., in the December 1993 *American Journal of Public Health.* "There are no easy answers to the question of how and when powerful drugs should be used among healthy people to prevent illnesses that may or may not ever occur," she says.

Rosenberg continues, "There has been a tendency to count the potential benefits of hormone supplements as real benefits, to discount potential risks and to prematurely extend use from high-risk to lower-risk women despite inadequate knowledge of the benefits and risks. The tendency by some physicians to routinely treat all recently menopausal women with supplements suggests a lack of consideration of the individual benefit-risk equation for each woman and of the alternatives." In light of the widespread and increasing prescription of hormone supplements by physicians in the United States—sales of just one estrogen product, Premarin, totaled $853 million in 1994 alone, according to the June 15, 1995, *Wall Street Journal*—Rosenberg and like-minded health care practitioners believe this is an appropriate time to reconsider how these drugs should be used and by whom.

Where Does the Medical Establishment Stand?

With all the dissension in the ranks of American physicians, what do professional medical associations advise their doctor members? The American College of Obstetricians and Gynecologists, for one, publishes technical bulletins for its physician members every few years. Its latest bulletin on HRT, published in 1992, summarizes the therapy with these words: "Hormone replacement therapy, although not suited to all patients, can confer health benefits, enhance quality of life and prolong life expectancy."

As for probable long-term health benefits, the bulletin uses "if" language: If estrogen reduces the probability of coronary heart disease and osteoporotic fractures, then it will generally increase life expectancy and may translate into better quality of life. But "if combination therapy does not provide as much protection against coronary heart disease as does unopposed estrogen, then women at high risk for breast cancer could actually have a decreased life expectancy," the guidelines state.

The American College of Physicians stated its position to its members in its 1992 Clinical Guidelines, published in the pages of the *Annals of Internal Medicine* (December 15, 1992), advising in general that "all women, regardless of race, should consider preventive hormone therapy." Speaking more specifically, the college noted that "hormone therapy should probably be recommended for women who have had a hysterectomy and for those with coronary heart disease or at high risk for coronary heart disease. For other women the best course for action is unclear."

These position statements will no doubt change as new research on HRT comes to light. Your doctor's position on HRT will be influenced by what she has seen in her practice, by what (and how much) she reads, by her medical specialty (statistically speaking, gynecologists embrace and prescribe HRT more often than general practitioners) and even by the opinions and concerns voiced by her patients. In other words, you do have a voice, and your opinions can and should count in the process of evaluating HRT.

■ The Decision-Making Continuum

Here's a chart designed to help you assess the benefits and risks of hormone replacement therapy. It is not meant to tell you whether to use HRT or not, but to help you identify relevant aspects of your personal medical history and clarify where you stand on the use of HRT after menopause. Based on what you have learned throughout this book concerning these issues, tick off those conditions or situations that apply to you. Some conditions are listed twice, indicating discrepancies in opinions in the medical field. Use this checklist as a jumping-off point for discussions about HRT between you and your health care practitioner.

Reasons NOT to take HRT

☐ Personal or family history of breast cancer
☐ Endometrial cancer
☐ History of thrombosis, including heart attacks or strokes caused by blood clots

▼

☐ Liver disease
☐ Impaired liver function
☐ Undiagnosed vaginal bleeding

Reasons MAYBE NOT to take HRT

☐ High blood pressure
☐ Gallbladder disease
☐ Diabetes mellitus
☐ Fibroids
☐ Migraines
☐ Endometriosis
☐ Seizure disorders
☐ Congestive heart failure
☐ Family history of very high blood cholesterol
☐ DES use by you or your mother

Reasons MAYBE to take HRT

☐ Average or moderate risk of osteoporosis
☐ Average or moderate risk of heart disease
☐ Mild to moderate menopausal symptoms
☐ Atrophic vaginitis
☐ Vaginal infections
☐ Urinary tract infections
☐ Alzheimer's disease

Reasons to take HRT

☐ High risk of osteoporosis
☐ High risk of heart disease
☐ Severe menopausal symptoms
☐ Atrophic vaginitis
☐ Frequent vaginal infections
☐ Frequent urinary tract infections

Determining Your Own
Benefit-Risk Ratio

So how do you decide? Admittedly it's no easy task. But we've devised some questions to help you focus on all that you've read in this book and see how it affects you. Use these questions to crystalize your feelings toward hormone replacement therapy and develop your own benefit-risk ratio.

• What is your view of menopause? Do you see it as a medical condition that needs treatment or a natural passage in life?

• Why are you considering HRT? Is it because your doctor advised you to, because you are experiencing menopause-related discomforts or because you are concerned about long-term health issues?

• Are you interested in short-term HRT or long-term HRT? Why? What would you like to achieve?

• Are you interested in nondrug or herbal alternatives to HRT? Why? What would you like to achieve?

• Are you interested in supplementing HRT with nondrug or alternative therapies? Why? What would you like to achieve?

• What is your personal risk of heart disease, osteoporosis and endometrial cancer? Are you at high risk, low risk, moderate risk for any of these conditions? If you are at high risk, what other therapies are available? What do you think of them? How do they compare to HRT? If you are at moderate or low risk, are there preventive steps that you should take instead of HRT, before beginning it, or in conjunction?

• What is your personal risk of breast cancer? How does this risk compare with your risk of heart disease, osteoporosis and endometrial cancer?

• Have you tried HRT in the past? Did you experience any side effects? Would you want to try a different HRT regimen? What side effects would you like to avoid?

• How much time do you want to invest in your health care? Many HRT alternatives require a large commitment in time and energy. Can you maintain a regular exercise regimen? Are you willing to maintain a healthy eating plan? Is your schedule so tight that you'd rather take hormone pills to possibly gain cardiovascular or osteoporotic protection than allot time for exercise and proper nutrition?

• How comfortable are you participating in the medical system? Are you more comfortable with the scientific (allopathic or osteopathic) medical approach, with its emphasis on medication and other interventions, or do you prefer a holistic or alternative form of medical care?

• What do you expect in terms of direction, advice and guidance from your practitioner? Do you want your health care practitioner to determine and direct your treatment and handle all the details? Do you want to be an equal partner in treatment decisions? Do you want to be kept abreast of all recent HRT research?

To this list add other questions or comments of your own.

There are no right or wrong answers. The key is to be honest. Evaluate your health, your desires, and then look at the evidence about HRT use as we know it today. With these thoughts and opinions, approach your health care practitioner and discuss HRT as it applies to you.

We wish we could say that everything you need to know about HRT lies within the covers of this book, but that would be a false promise. The fact is that everything you need to know has not yet come to light. Experts disagree about the benefits and risks of hormone replacement; scientific studies give contradictory results.

In the interim you have to make your decision with less-than-perfect information. As you weigh hormone replacement therapy, remember that your decision cannot be made on purely statistical grounds. You are unique. Your choice must reflect your personal concerns, your personal risks—keeping in mind the subtle differences between treatment and prevention and your goals for your health throughout your life.

Acupressure Institute
1533 Shattuck Ave.
Berkeley, CA 94709
510-845-1059
> Provides free *Hands-on Health Care Catalog* of books, videos and acupressure tools.

American Academy of Family Physicians
8880 Ward Pkwy.
Kansas City, MO 64114
816-333-9700
800-274-2237
> Provides names of family physicians in your area.

American Association of Acupuncture and
    Oriental Medicine
4101 Lake Boone Trail, Suite 201
Raleigh, NC 27607
> Provides national referral directory of members who meet acceptable standards of competency. Available by mail only for $8 prepaid.

American Association of Naturopathic Physicians
2366 Eastlake Ave., E., Suite 322
Seattle, WA 98102
206-323-7610

> Provides national referral directory of all U.S. members and information brochure about naturopathic medicine for $5 prepaid.

American Botanical Council
P.O. Box 201660
Austin, TX 78720
512-331-8868

> Publishes *HerbalGram* magazine and booklets on herbs. Offers reprints of scientific articles. Sells hard-to-locate books on herbalism.

American Cancer Society
1599 Clifton Rd., N.E.
Atlanta, GA 30329
404-320-3333
800-ACS-2345

> Publishes free material about cancer prevention and treatment.

American College of Nurse-Midwives
818 Connecticut Ave., N.W., Suite 900
Washington, DC 20006
202-728-9860

> Provides listings of nurse-midwives by state and pamphlets and brochures.

American College of Obstetricians and Gynecologists
409 12th St., S.W.
Washington, DC 20024
202-638-5577

> Publishes free patient information pamphlets. Provides lists of board-certified physicians in your geographic area.

American Dietetic Association
216 W. Jackson Blvd., Suite 800
Chicago, IL 60606
312-899-0040

> Provides information on nutrition.

American Heart Association
7272 Greenville Ave.
Dallas, TX 75231
214-373-6300

> Publishes materials on heart disease prevention and treatment.

American Herbalists Guild
P.O. Box 1683
Sequel, CA 95073

> Provides directory of schools and teachers of medical herbalism in the United States.

Biofeedback Certification Institute of America
10200 W. 44th Ave., Suite 304
Wheat Ridge, CO 80033
303-420-2902

> Runs the major certification program for biofeedback practitioners. Provides information about certified local practitioners.

Boston Women's Health Book Collective
Box 192
West Somerville, MA 02114
617-625-0271

Medical consumer/membership organization. Maintains consumer health library open to public. Publishes books and brochures on women's health issues. Send a business-size, self-addressed, stamped envelope for a list of publications, services and current activities.

Cancer Information Service of the
National Cancer Institute
NCI/NIH, Bldg. 31, 10A24
9000 Rockville Pike
Bethesda, MD 20892
800-4-CANCER

Provides free cancer information service. Staffed by trained counselors. Offers details on 150 types of cancer, referrals to hospitals, support groups and information on financial aid.

Center for Medical Consumers
237 Thompson St.
New York, NY 10012
212-674-7105

Provides a medical library and publishes *HealthFacts,* a newsletter that clearly presents controversial health care issues.

A Friend Indeed
Box 1710
Champlain, NY 12919-1710
514-843-5730

Monthly newsletter. Provides information about the latest research on menopause and other health topics for women.

HERS (Hysterectomy Educational Resources and
   Services) Foundation
422 Bryn Mawr Ave.
Bala Cynwyd, PA 19004
610-667-7757
   Offers a quarterly newsletter on hysterectomy-related issues,
   referral list of doctors for second opinions, and guidelines
   on developing a local support group.

Hot Flash: Newsletter for Midlife and Older Women
National Action Forum for Midlife and Older Women
P.O. Box 816
Stony Brook, NY 11790-0816
   Provides information on the health needs of and resources
   for older women.

Menopause News
800-241-MENO
   Newsletter with information on latest research and
   developments in treating menopausal symptoms.

Menotimes
1108 Irwin St.
San Rafael, CA 94901
415-459-5430
   Quarterly journal for consumers and health care practitioners interested in holistic practices and alternative
   therapies to HRT. Available for $30/year.

Midlife Women's Support Group
c/o Rose Langfelder
30 Third Ave.
Brooklyn, NY 11217
718-875-1420

> Local support group for women over age 40 in the
> Brooklyn area. Holds free workshops periodically on
> any topic related to midlife.

National Center for Homeopathy
801 N. Fairfax St., Suite 306
Alexandria, VA 22314
703-548-7790

> Provides a packet to consumers for $6, which includes
> general information and the annual directory of
> homeopathic practitioners and study groups.

National Commission for the Certification
    of Acupuncturists
1424 16th St., N.W., Suite 501
Washington, DC 20036
202-232-1404

> Provides state list of certified acupuncturists for $3 prepaid.
> Send your request in writing.

National Osteoporosis Foundation
1150 17th St., N.W., Suite 500
Washington, DC 20036
202-223-2226

> Publishes pamphlets and offers copies of research articles
> on the subject of osteoporosis.

National Self-Help Clearinghouse
25 W. 43rd St., Room 620
New York, NY 10036
212-642-2944
FAX 212-642-1956

> Publishes the newsletter *The Self-Help Reporter*. Offers
> referrals to national support groups. Send a business-size,
> self-addressed, stamped envelope with the name or topic
> of the support group for which you're looking.

National Women's Health Network
514 10th St., N.W., Suite 400
Washington, DC 20004
202-347-1140

> Offers packets of resource materials on general or specific
> topics. Available for $8. Write for a free directory of topics
> and a one-page brief on your particular health concerns.

National Women's Health Resource Center
2440 M St., N.W., Suite 325
Washington, DC 20037
202-293-6045

> Publishes a newsletter on current women's health issues.
> Special report addressing menopause and hormone
> replacement available by mail only for $2 prepaid.

North American Menopause Society
University Hospitals of Cleveland
Department of OB/GYN
11100 Euclid Ave.
Cleveland, OH 44106
216-844-3334

> Provides information on menopause. Offers lists of meno-
> pause treatment centers and free quarterly newsletter.

Women—Midlife and Menopause
Clara Wood Anthony
737 Morrison Dr.
Greenbelt, MD 20770

> Local support group. Provides information and referrals on midlife changes and menopause for women in the Greenbelt, Maryland, area. Offers help in starting a local support group. Packet of group materials, $5.

Resource Books of Interest

Alternative Medicine Yellow Pages. Future Medicine Publishing (Puyallup, Wash.: Future Medicine Publishing, 1994).

> Lists national organizations and local chapters of alternative practitioners.

Medical & Health Information Directory, 1994–95. Karen Boyden, ed. (Detroit: Gale Research, Inc., 1994).

The Official ABMS Directory of Board-Certified Medical Specialists, 1995. (New Providence, N.J.: Marquis Who's Who, 1994).

> Lists U.S. physicians who are board certified in their medical specialties.

GLOSSARY

Absolute contraindications: Situations or medical conditions that prohibit the use of HRT.

Acupressure: Healing art in which the fingers are used to apply pressure to specific sites on the body to treat illness and restore health.

Acupuncture: Healing art in which thin needles are inserted under the skin at specific sites on the body to treat illness and restore health.

Adrenal glands: Glands alongside the kidneys that produce many hormones, including epinephrine (adrenaline), androstenedione (later converted into estrone), testosterone, mineralocorticoids and glucocorticoids.

Amenorrhea: Lack of menstruation; abnormal cessation of menstrual cycle.

Androgen: Substance (such as a hormone) that produces masculine characteristics in the body.

Androstenedione: Hormone produced by the adrenal glands that fatty tissue in the body converts to estrone.

Angina: Chest pain caused by insufficient blood flow to the heart.

Angiotensin: Chemical that causes blood vessels to narrow.

Anise: Phytoestrogenic herb sometimes used to relieve menopausal discomforts.

Antihypertensives: Drugs used to lower blood pressure.

Artificial menopause: Menopause caused by surgical removal of the ovaries.

Aspiration endometrial biopsy: Endometrial biopsy made with a suction instrument.

Atrophic: Degenerative.

Atrophic vaginitis: Shrinkage, drying and lessening elasticity of vaginal tissues after menopause; can cause discomfort during sexual intercourse and lead to more frequent vaginal infections.

Atrophy: To wither, degenerate.

Baseline: First test to which later ones are compared.

Bile: Thick, amber-colored liquid manufactured by the liver, stored in the gallbladder and discharged in the digestive tract; breaks down fats to aid digestion.

Biofeedback: Psychological therapy that uses the conscious mind to control involuntary body functions such as respiration, heartbeat and body temperature.

Biphasic pills: Type of birth control pill that contains a steady dose of estrogen throughout the cycle but varying doses of progestin.

Biphosphonates: Class of drugs that can prevent bone loss.

Black cohosh: Phytoestrogenic herb sometimes used to relieve hot flashes and vaginal dryness.

Bone mass: Total amount of bone tissue.

Bone resorption: Process by which bones dissolve and lose calcium.

Breakthrough bleeding: Unplanned, abnormal uterine bleeding between menstrual periods.

Buccal estrogen: Estrogen administered by means of a tablet placed inside your mouth, against the cheek, so that the estrogen is absorbed through the mucous membranes into the bloodstream.

Calcitonin: Hormone that decreases calcium in the bloodstream and is thought to help bones absorb calcium.

Calcium to creatinine ratio: Urine test to determine how quickly bone mass is being lost.

Cerebrovascular accident: Stroke.

Certified nurse-midwife: Registered nurse who has completed graduate training in women's health, obstetrical care and gynecological care and has passed an extensive credentialing examination.

Cervix: Bottom of the uterus that extends into the vagina.

Chamomile: Herb sometimes used as a relaxant.

Clonidine: Antihypertensive drug; may relieve hot flashes.

Collagen: Protein that provides structural support for bone, skin, cartilage and connective tissue.

Combination therapy: Form of HRT in which a woman takes progestin in addition to one of the forms of estrogen.

Complete fractures: Breaks involving the entire width of a bone.

Compression fractures: Breaks that collapse the bone.

Conjugated equine estrogen: Estrogen in pill form derived from the urine of pregnant mares.

Continuous combined therapy: Form of HRT in which a small amount of progestin is taken along with estrogen every day of the month.

Continuous sequential therapy: Form of HRT in which a woman takes estrogen continuously, every day of the month. Progestin is taken for 12 to 14 days throughout a month, from day 12 through day 25.

Cornified cells: Type of cells that develop on the surface of the vagina after estrogen levels have been depleted for several months or more.

Corpus luteum: Ruptured follicle's scar tissue that temporarily manufactures progesterone.

Cortical bone: Dense and hard tissue; outer layer of bone.

Cyclic AMP (cAMP): Body chemical involved in nervous system, hormone and cell functions.

Cyclic combined therapy: Form of HRT in which a woman takes estrogen and low-dosage progestin for 25 days each month.

Cyclic sequential therapy: Form of HRT in which a woman takes estrogen for 21 days or 25 days of the month, with progestin taken along with the estrogen for the last 10 or 14 days.

Dilatation and curettage (D&C): Surgical procedure that dilates (widens) the cervix so the physician can scrape and remove endometrium with a curette (spoon-shaped instrument).

Diuretic: A drug that promotes the production and discharge of urine.

D.O.: Doctor of osteopathy.

Dong quai: Phytoestrogenic herb sometimes used to treat hot flashes.

Dual-energy x-ray absorptiometry: Test that measures the amount of bone tissue in the wrist, arm, spine, hip or thighbone.

Dual-photon absorptiometry: Test that measures density of the spine, hip or thighbone.

Ectopic pregnancy: Life-threatening pregnancy in which a fertilized egg implants itself in a fallopian tube instead of the uterus.

Embolism: Blockage of a blood vessel caused by an embolus.

Embolus: Blood clot, object, bit of tissue or gas in a blood vessel.

Endocrine glands: Glands that manufacture hormones and release them into the bloodstream.

Endocrine system: Network of glands that manufacture hormones and release them into the bloodstream.

Endocrinologist: M.D. or D.O. specializing in the treatment of hormonal disorders, including problems related to menopause as well as diabetes, pituitary diseases and sexual problems.

Endometrial biopsy: Medical procedure in which a small tissue sample is removed from the endometrium (uterine lining) to look for the presence of abnormal cells.

Endometrial hyperplasia: See **hyperplasia.**

Endometrial sampling: See **endometrial biopsy.**

Endometriosis: Condition in which cells from the endometrium (uterine lining) migrate outside the uterus and grow on other organs in the abdomen.

Endometrium: Lining of the uterus.

ERT: See **estrogen replacement therapy.**

Esterified estrogen: Form of natural estrogen used in HRT.

Estradiol: Most potent form of estrogen; produced by the ovaries.

Estragel: Name for an estrogen gel used in Europe. Estrogen is delivered into the bloodstream through the skin by means of gel rubbed on the abdomen.

Estriol: A weak estrogen produced in the female body.

Estrogen: One of several hormones that control the reproductive process in the female body. The three estrogens are estradiol, estrone and estriol.

Estrogen replacement therapy (ERT): Medical treatment to replace some of the estrogen lost after menopause; a form of hormone replacement therapy.

Estrone: Low-level estrogen produced in the body's fatty tissues.

Estropipate: Synthetic estrogen used in HRT.

Etridronate: A biphosphonate; used to treat osteoporosis.

Fallopian tubes: Two thin tubes that capture eggs as they leave the ovaries and channel them to the uterus.

False unicorn: Phytoestrogenic herb sometimes used to treat menopausal symptoms.

Family practitioner: M.D. or D.O. specializing in the total health care of the individual (woman, man, adult or child) and the family.

Fennel: Phytoestrogenic herb sometimes used to treat menopausal symptoms.

Fibroids: Noncancerous growths in uterine muscle tissue.

Flavonoids: Colorful and aromatic compounds found in fruit that are weak phytoestrogens; also known as bioflavonoids.

Follicle-stimulating hormone (FSH): Hormone released by the pituitary to stimulate the ovaries to produce estrogen and encourage the egg follicles in the ovaries to mature.

Formication: Sensation of something crawling on the skin; a vasomotor symptom of menopause.

Fractures: Breaks.

FSH: See **follicle-stimulating hormone.**

FSH test: Blood test that measures the amount of follicle-stimulating hormone; used to make a diagnosis of menopause. Levels greater than 30 IU/ml indicate that menopause is imminent; readings over 40 IU/ml mark indicate the onset of menopause.

Gall: See **bile.**

Genitourinary symptoms: Symptoms occurring months or years after menopause in response to low estrogen levels; includes more frequent urination, vaginal dryness, vaginal infections and urinary tract infections.

Ginseng: Phytoestrogenic herb sometimes used to treat menopausal discomforts.

Gonadotropin-releasing hormones: Hormones released by the hypothalamus that tell the pituitary to release one of two gonadotropins: follicle-stimulating hormone and luteinizing hormone.

Gonadotropins: Hormones that cause the ovaries and testes to act.

Gynecologist: M.D. or D.O. trained in the health and proper functioning of the female reproductive system (gynecology).

HDL: See **high-density lipoprotein.**

Herbalist: Practitioner skilled in the art of herbal medicine; compounds herbal mixtures made from plants.

High-density lipoprotein (HDL): So-called good cholesterol that helps to escort cholesterol from the body. High levels are linked with reduced risk for heart disease.

Hirsutism: Excessive hair growth on the upper lip or chin.

Homeopathic physician: M.D. or D.O. with additional training in homeopathy.

Homeopathic practitioner: M.D., D.O., nurse practitioner, nurse-midwife, physician assistant, licensed acupuncturist, naturopathic physician or veterinarian who practices homeopathy.

Homeopathy: System of medicine that treats illness by using natural medicines that stimulate a person's own healing powers while avoiding harmful side effects.

Hormone replacement therapy (HRT): Medical treatment to replace some of the estrogen and progesterone lost after menopause.

Hormones: Naturally occurring chemicals in one part of body that produce physical effects in another part of the body.

Hot flashes: Menopausal symptoms characterized by a sensation of intense warmth and a pink flush in the head, neck and upper body that can last from a few seconds to an hour.

Hot flush: Another term for hot flash.

HRT: See **hormone replacement therapy.**

Hyperplasia: Proliferation of cells in the uterine lining that can lead to uterine cancer.

Hypertension: High blood pressure.

Hypothalamus: Small but powerful gland in the brain that oversees the reproductive endocrine system as well as other body functions.

Hysterectomy: Surgical removal of the uterus.

Hysteroscopy: Procedure in which a flexible fiberoptic viewing tube is inserted inside the uterus so the doctor can examine the uterus and/or take tissue samples.

Implanted subcutaneous estrogen pellets: Estrogen administered by means of pellets or capsules surgically implanted under the skin.

Incomplete fractures: Breaks that don't go all the way through a bone.

International unit (IU): Unit of measurement.

Internist: M.D. or D.O. specializing in the diagnosis and non-surgical treatment of disease, especially those of adults.

Kegel exercises: Exercises that strengthen muscles that control urination; also called pubococcygeus exercises, after the muscles affected.

LDL: See **low-density lipoprotein.**

LH: See **luteinizing hormone.**

Licorice: Phytoestrogenic herb sometimes used to treat hot flashes.

Lipids: Greasy substances such as fatty acids and waxes; stored in the body for use as energy reserves.

Local: Pertaining to one specific area of the body.

Low-density lipoprotein (LDL): So-called bad cholesterol. High levels of LDL cholesterol have been linked with increased risk for heart disease.

Luteinizing hormone (LH): Gonadotropin hormone that causes ovulation.

Mastalgia: Breast tenderness or pain.

M.D.: Doctor of medicine.

Mediators: Substances made of fatty acids that help hormones carry out their jobs.

Medroxyprogesterone acetate: Form of progestin often used in HRT.

Megesterol acetate: Form of progestin sometimes used in HRT.

Menarche: First menstrual period; signifies the beginning of menstruation and the start of the reproductive years.

Menopause: Normal and complete cessation of menstrual cycles; in everyday usage, the months before and years after the last period.

Methyldopa: Antihypertensive drug; may reduce hot flashes.

Microgram (mcg): Unit of measurement; one-millionth of a gram.

Micronized estradiol: Form of estrogen sold in pills.

Monophasic pills: Type of birth control pills that contain the same amount of estrogen and progestin in each pill throughout the cycle.

Motherwort: Herb sometimes used by menopausal women to relieve palpitations that accompany hot flashes.

Natural estrogens: Type of drug using estrogens that are naturally occurring and are similar to the estrogens made in the human body.

Natural progesterone: Type of drug using progesterone that is naturally occurring and similar to the progesterone made in the body.

Naturopathy: Healing art that emphasizes using the body's natural healing forces.

N.D.: Doctor of naturopathic medicine; practices naturopathy.

Nocturia: Excessive urination at night.

Norethindrone: Type of progestin used in birth control pills.

Norgestrel: Type of progestin used in birth control pills.

Nurse practitioner: Registered nurse with additional graduate training.

Obstetrician: M.D. or D.O. trained in all aspects of pregnancy and childbirth (obstetrics).

Oophorectomy: Surgical removal of the ovaries.

Opiates: Chemicals that induce rest and quiet uneasiness.

Oral contraceptive: Birth control pill.

Oral estrogen: Estrogen in pill form.

Osteopathy: Practice of medicine that uses all the usual techniques of drugs, surgery and radiation, but looks more at the links between the organs and the musculoskeletal system.

Osteopenia: Low bone mass.

Osteoporosis: Condition in which bones gradually lose their mineral content, becoming porous, thin and fragile.

Ovary: One of two female endocrine glands that contain unfertilized egg cells; produces the hormones estrogen, progesterone and testosterone.

Ovulation: Release of an egg from the ovary.

Paget's disease: Disease characterized by excessive bone destruction and poor bone structure.

Pamidronate: A biphosphonate; used to treat osteoporosis.

Parathyroid hormone: Hormone that works to maintain an even amount of calcium in the blood.

Parathyroids: Four small glands, attached alongside the thyroid, that manufacture parathyroid hormone, which helps to keep the level of blood calcium normal.

Pelvic inflammatory disease: Serious bacterial infection of the uterus, fallopian tubes and/or uterus.

Perimenopause: Years immediately before menopause.

Phlebitis: Inflammation of a vein due to presence of blood clot.

Phytoestrogens: Chemicals that the body converts into estrogen; also known as plant estrogens. Foods high in phytoestrogens include soy products (soybeans, tofu, miso), papaya and yams. Lesser amounts can be found in apples, brown rice, carrots, green beans, peas, potatoes, red beans, sesame seeds, whole wheat and rye.

Pill, the: Abbreviated term for birth control pill.

Pituitary: Pebble-sized endocrine gland that works in conjunction with the hypothalamus to regulate hormone production in the body.

Plant estrogens: See **phytoestrogens.**

Platelets: Small cells in the blood.

Postmenopause: After menopause.

Premature menopause: Menopause before age 40, regardless of the reason.

Progesterone: Female sex hormone produced by the ovaries during the second half of the menstrual cycle.

Progesterone challenge test: Used to determine whether irregular menstrual periods or hyperplasia is caused by insufficient progesterone levels.

Progestin: Synthetic or man-made progesterone.

Progestin-only pills: Type of birth control pills that contain small amounts of progestin and no estrogen at all; dubbed "minipills."

Prophylactic: Preventive.

Prostaglandin: A chemical mediator that causes contractions in the uterus.

Puberty: In females the time during which a girl's body sexually matures, making her capable of reproduction.

Pubococcygeus exercises: See **Kegel exercises.**

Quantitative computed tomography (CT scan or QCT scan): Test to measure trabecular bone within the vertebrae and create a 3-D image of the spine.

Radiographic absorptiometry (RA): X-ray taken of the hand to determine bone density, detect fractures and help the health care practitioner diagnose osteoporosis.

Red clover: Weakly phytoestrogenic herb sometimes used to treat menopausal symptoms.

Relative contraindications: Situations or medical conditions under which HRT should be used with great care and medical supervision.

Salmon calcitonin: Drug to prevent further bone loss in women with osteoporosis.

Sedatives: Drugs that decrease activity, relieve anxiety and produce calm.

Single-phase pills: Type of birth control pills that contain the same amount of estrogen and progestin in each pill throughout the cycle.

Single-photon absorptiometry: Test that determines the bone density of the wrist or heel.

Sodium fluoride: Drug used to treat osteoporosis.

Surgical menopause: Menopause caused by surgical removal of the ovaries.

Synthetic estrogens: Pharmaceutically produced estrogen, synthesized using petroleum-based chemicals; more potent than natural estrogens.

Synthetic progestin: Type of drug that tends to be more potent than natural progesterones.

Systemic: Pertaining to or affecting the entire body.

T₃ (triiodothyronine): Thyroid hormone that affects how well cells consume oxygen, thus affecting the body's metabolic functions and its growth and development.

T₄ (thyroxine): Thyroid hormone that affects how well cells consume oxygen, thus affecting the body's metabolic functions and its growth and development.

Testosterone: Androgen (male hormone) produced in small amounts by the ovaries.

Thromboembolism: Blood vessel blocked by a blood clot.

Thrombophlebitis: Blood clot and inflammation in a deep vein, such as in a leg.

Thrombosis: Condition characterized by blood clots in a blood vessel.

Thrombus: Blood clot.

Thyroid gland: Organ located just below the voice box that secretes three hormones: T₃ (triiodothyronine) and T₄ (thyroxine), which affect how well cells consume oxygen, thus affecting the growth and development of every part of the body, and calcitonin, a hormone that decreases calcium in the bloodstream and is thought to help bones absorb calcium.

Total hysterectomy: Surgical removal of the uterus and cervix.

Trabecular bone: Porous bone tissue.

Tranquilizers: Drugs that calm, lessen anxiety and tension and induce drowsiness.

Transdermal estrogen: Estrogen administered by means of an adhesive patch applied to the skin.

Triphasic pills: Type of birth control pills that vary the amount of both estrogen and progestin during the month.

Ultrasound: Imaging of organs and structures deep inside the body made with high-frequency sound waves.

Unopposed estrogen: Estrogen given alone (without either natural or synthetic progestin). Generally, unopposed estrogen is prescribed only for women without a uterus; in women with a uterus, unopposed estrogen increases the risk of hyperplasia.

Urethra: Tube that drains urine from the bladder.

Urinary hydroxyproline: Urine test to determine bone loss and the breakdown of other tissue.

Uterus: Female organ composed of muscle and glandular tissue; the womb.

Vagina: Resilient, muscular tract that extends from the uterus to the vulva, the outer genitals of the female body.

Vaginal estrogen cream: Estrogen administered by means of an applicator that dispenses a measured amount of cream into the vagina.

Vaginal ring implant: Estrogen delivered by means of a ring inserted in the vagina and left there to slowly release estradiol; not yet available in the United States.

Vaginitis: Vaginal infection.

Vasomotor symptoms: Menopausal symptoms that relate to the nerves and muscles that open and close blood vessels; include hot flashes and night sweats.

Withdrawal bleeding: Regular uterine bleeding that occurs in some women taking certain combination forms of HRT; similar to a menstrual period.

Womb: See **uterus.**

Books and Booklets

American College of Obstetricians and Gynecologists. *Hormone Replacement Therapy.* Technical Bulletin Number 166, April 1992.

Bauer, Cathryn. *Acupressure for Everybody: Gentle, Effective Relief for More Than 100 Common Ailments.* New York: Holt, 1991.

Bonk, Melinda, ed. *Alternative Medicine: The Definitive Guide.* Puyallup, Wash.: Future Medicine Publishing, 1994.

Boston Women's Health Book Collective. *The New Our Bodies, Ourselves.* New York: Simon & Schuster, 1992.

Carr, Bruce R., M.D., and Jean D. Wilson, M.D. "Disorders of the Ovary and Female Reproductive Tract." In *Harrison's Principles of Internal Medicine,* 12th ed. Edited by Kurt J. Isselbacher, M.D., et al. New York: McGraw-Hill, 1994.

Castleman, Michael. *The Healing Herbs: The Ultimate Guide to the Curative Powers of Nature's Medicines.* Emmaus, Pa.: Rodale Press, 1991.

Cherry, Sheldon H., M.D., and Carolyn D. Runowicz, M.D. *The Menopause Book: A Guide to Health and Well-Being for Women After Forty.* New York: Macmillan, 1994.

Cobb, Janine O'Leary. *Understanding Menopause: Answers & Advice for Women in the Prime of Life.* New York: Penguin Books, 1993.

Coney, Sandra. *The Menopause Industry: How the Medical Establishment Exploits Women.* Alameda, Calif.: Hunter House, 1994.

Gardner, Joy. *The New Healing Yourself: Natural Remedies for Adults and Children.* Freedom, Calif.: The Crossing Press, 1989.

Greenwood, Sadja, M.D. *Menopause Naturally, Updated: Preparing for the Second Half of Life.* Volcano, Calif.: Volcano Press, 1992.

Heaney, Robert P., M.D., and M. Janet Barger-Lux. *Calcium and Common Sense.* New York: Doubleday, 1988.

Inlander, Charles B., and the staff of the People's Medical Society. *The Consumer's Medical Desk Reference.* New York: Hyperion, 1995.

Ito, Dee. *Without Estrogen: Natural Remedies for Menopause and Beyond.* New York: Carol Southern Books, 1994.

Jovanovic, Lois, M.D., with Suzanne Levert. *A Woman Doctor's Guide to Menopause.* New York: Hyperion, 1993.

Jovanovic, Lois, M.D., and Genell J. Subak-Sharpe, M.S. *Hormones: The Woman's Answerbook.* New York: Ivy Books, 1987.

Landau, Carol, Ph.D., Michele G. Cyr, M.D., and Anne W. Moulton, M.D. *The Complete Book of Menopause: Every Woman's Guide to Good Health.* New York: G. P. Putnam's Sons, 1994.

Lark, Susan M. *The Menopause Self-Help Book.* Berkeley, Calif.: Celestial Arts Publishing, 1990.

Lockie, Andrew, M.D., and Nicola Geddes, M.D. *The Women's Guide to Homeopathy.* New York: St. Martin's Press, 1994.

Mishell, Daniel R., Jr., M.D. "Menopause." In *Conn's Current Therapy 1995.* Edited by Robert E. Rakel, M.D. Philadelphia: W. B. Saunders, 1995.

Murray, Michael, N.D., and Joseph Pizzorno, N.D. *The Encyclopedia of Natural Medicine.* Rocklin, Calif.: Prima, 1991.

Nachtigall, Lila, M.D., and Joan Rattner Heilman. *Estrogen: The Facts Can Change Your Life.* Revised and expanded. New York: Harper & Row, 1991.

Notelovitz, Morris, M.D., Ph.D., and Diana Tonnessen. *Menopause and Midlife Health.* New York: St. Martin's Press, 1993.

Ojeda, Linda, Ph.D. *Menopause Without Medicine.* Alameda, Calif.: Hunter House, 1992.

Perry, Susan, and Katherine O'Hanlan, M.D. *Natural Menopause: The Complete Guide to a Woman's Most Misunderstood Passage.* Reading, Mass.: Addison-Wesley, 1992.

Shapiro, Howard I., M.D. *The New Birth Control Book.* New York: Prentice Hall, 1988.

Smith, Kristen E., M.D., and Howard L. Judd, M.D. "Menopause and Postmenopause." In *Current Obstetric and Gynecologic Diagnosis and Treatment,* 8th ed. Edited by Alan H. DeCherney, M.D., and Martin L. Pernoll, M.D. Norwalk, Conn.: Appleton & Lange, 1994.

Utian, Wulf H., M.D., Ph.D., and Ruth S. Jacobowitz. *Managing Your Menopause.* New York: Simon & Schuster, 1990.

Winikoff, Beverly, M.D., M.P.H., Suzanne Wymelenberg, and the editors of Consumer Reports Books. *The Contraceptive Handbook: A Guide to Safe and Effective Choices.* Yonkers, N.Y.: Consumer Reports Books, 1992.

Wyngaarden, James B., M.D, et al., eds. "The Menopause and Postmenopausal Years." In *Cecil Textbook of Medicine,* 19th edition. Philadelphia: W. B. Saunders, 1992.

Articles

Aloia, John F., M.D., et al. "Calcium Supplementation With and Without Hormone Replacement Therapy to Prevent Post-menopausal Bone Loss." *Annals of Internal Medicine* 120, no. 2 (January 15, 1994): 97-103.

American College of Physicians. "Guidelines for Counseling Postmenopausal Women About Preventive Hormone Therapy." *Annals of Internal Medicine* 117, no. 12 (December 15, 1992): 1038-41.

Bachmann, Gloria A., M.D. "Estrogen-Androgen Therapy for Sexual and Emotional Well-Being." *Female Patient* 18, no. 7 (July 1993): 15-24.

Barrett-Connor, Elizabeth, M.D. "Risks and Benefits of Replacement Estrogen." *Annual Review of Medicine* 43 (1992): 239-51.

Barrett-Connor, Elizabeth, M.D., and Trudy L. Bush, Ph.D., M.H.S. "Estrogen and Coronary Heart Disease in Women." *Journal of the American Medical Association* 265, no. 14 (April 10, 1991): 1861-67.

Bewley, S., and T. H. Bewley. Drug Dependence With Estrogen Replacement Therapy." *Lancet* 339 (February 1, 1992): 290-91.

Brody, Jane E. "Depression at Menopause: Sorting Out the Myths," *New York Times,* 21 September 1994, sec. C, p. 10.

———. "New Therapy for Menopause Reduces Risk," *New York Times,* 18 November 1994, sec. A, p. 1.

Byrjalsen, Inger, M.S., et al. "Role of Cigarette Smoking on the Postmenopausal Endometrium During Sequential Estrogen and Progestogen Therapy." *Obstetrics & Gynecology* 81, no. 6 (June 1993): 1016-1021.

Colditz, Graham A., M.B., B.S., et al. "The Use of Estrogens and Progestins and the Risk of Breast Cancer in Postmenopausal Women." *New England Journal of Medicine* 332, no. 24 (June 15, 1995): 1589-93.

DiSaia, Philip J., M.D. "Hormone Replacement Therapy in Patients With Breast Cancer." *Cancer* 71, no. 2 (February 15, 1993): 1490-1500.

"Drug Update: Hormone Replacement." *Internal Medicine News* 28, no. 11 (June 1, 1995): 25.

"ERT: Current Guidelines for Education and Counseling." *Journal of Gerontological Nursing* 16, no. 10 (October 1990): 6-11.

Ettinger, Bruce, M.D., and Deborah Grady, M.D. "The Waning Effect of Postmenopausal Estrogen Therapy on Osteoporosis." *New England Journal of Medicine* 329, no. 16 (October 14, 1993): 1192-93.

Falkeborn, Margareta, M.D., et al. "Hormone Replacement Therapy and the Risk of Stroke." *Archives of Internal Medicine* 153, no. 10 (May 21, 1993): 1201-9.

Fantl, J. Andrew, M.D., et al. "Estrogen Therapy in the Management of Urinary Incontinence in Postmenopausal Women: A Meta-Analysis. First Report of the Hormones and Urogenital Therapy Committee." *Obstetrics & Gynecology* 83, no. 1 (January 1994): 12-18.

Finucaine, Fanchon F., M.H.S., et al. "Decreased Risk of Stroke Among Postmenopausal Hormone Users." *Archives of Internal Medicine* 153, no. 1 (January 11, 1993): 73-79.

Gambrell, R. Don, Jr., M.D. "Update on Hormone Replacement Therapy." *American Family Physician* 46, no. 5 (November 1992): 87S-96S.

Grady, Deborah, M.D., M.P.H., et al. "Hormone Therapy to Prevent Disease and Prolong Life in Postmenopausal Women." *Annals of Internal Medicine* 117, no. 12 (December 12, 1992): 1016-37.

Hemminki, Elina, M.D., and Sinikka Shivo, M.P.H. "A Review of Postmenopausal Hormone Therapy Recommendations: Potential for Selection Bias." *Obstetrics & Gynecology* 82, no. 6 (December 1993): 1021-28.

Jacobs, J. S., and F. E. Loeffler. "Postmenopausal Hormone Replacement Therapy." *British Medical Journal* 305, no. 6866 (December 5, 1992): 1403-8.

Johannes, Catherine B., et al. "Longitudinal Patterns and Correlates of Hormone Replacement Therapy Use in Middle-Aged Women." *American Journal of Epidemiology* 140, no. 5 (September 1, 1994): 439-452.

Kolata, Gina. "Heart Ills and High Cholesterol May Not Be Linked in Old Age." *New York Times,* 2 November 1994, sec. C, p. 12.

Kubetin, Sally Koch. "Estrogen's Cardiac Benefit Waits for Randomized Support." *Internal Medicine News & Cardiology News* (November 1, 1994): 15.

Maddox, Marjorie A., Ed.D., R.N.C. "Women at Midlife: Hormone Replacement Therapy." *Nursing Clinics of North America* 27, no. 4 (December 1992): 959-69.

"Male Hormones Can Improve Sexual Function During Menopause." *Modern Medicine* 62 (January 1994): 36.

Marchant, Douglas J., M.D. "Estrogen Replacement Therapy After Breast Cancer." *Cancer* 71, no. 3 (March 15, 1993): 2169-76.

Marshburn, Paul B., M.D., and Bruce R. Carr, M.D. "Hormone Replacement Therapy: Protection Against the Consequences of Menopause." *Postgraduate Medicine* 92, no. 4 (September 15, 1992): 145-159.

Mestel, Rosie. "Can Estrogen Fend Off Alzheimer's?" *New Scientist* (November 20, 1993): 10.

Newman, Anthony. "Estrogen Benefits 'Many Years After Menopause.'" *Family Practice News* 23, no. 5 (March 1, 1993): 9.

Paganini-Hill, Annlia, and Victor W. Henderson. "Estrogen Deficiency and Risk of Alzheimer's Disease in Women." *American Journal of Epidemiology* 140, no. 3 (August 1, 1994): 256-61.

Parent-Stevens, Louise, Pharm.D. "Hormonal Replacement Therapy." *NARD Journal* 115, no. 6 (June 1993): 51-55.

Pass, David A., Pharm.D. "Estrogen Replacement: Its Role in Prevention and Treatment of Osteoporosis." *American Druggist* 208, no. 2 (July 1993): 47-51.

Pierce, Calvin. "HRT Benefits Worth the Potential Risks." *Internal Medicine News & Cardiology News* (September 1, 1994): 30.

Prince, Richard L., M.D., et al. "Prevention of Postmenopausal Osteoporosis." *New England Journal of Medicine* 325, no. 17 (October 24, 1991): 1189-95.

Rosenberg, Lynn, Sc.D. "Hormone Replacement Therapy: The Need for Reconsideration." *American Journal of Public Health* 83, no. 12 (December 1993): 1670-73.

Rudy, David R., M.D. "Hormone Replacement Therapy: How to Select the Best Preparation and Regimen." *Postgraduate Medicine* 88, no. 8 (December 1990): 157-164.

Saleh, AbdelAziz A., M.D., Ph.D., et al. "Thrombosis and Hormone Replacement Therapy in Postmenopausal Women." *American Journal of Obstetrics and Gynecology* 169, no. 6 (December 1993): 1554-1557.

Scalley, Erin K., B.S., and Janet B. Henrich, M.D. "An Overview of Estrogen Replacement Therapy in Postmenopausal Women." *Journal of Women's Health* 2, no. 3 (fall 1993): 289-294.

Scheck, Anne. "Unopposed Estrogen: Rethinking the Risks and Benefits." *Obstetrics/Gynecology News* 28, no. 23: 1.

Schiff, Isaac, M.D. "Keys to Balancing the Risks and Benefits of Estrogen Therapy for Postmenopausal Women." *Modern Medicine* 61, no. 1 (January 1993): 72-93.

Semla, Todd P., M.S., Pharm. D., and Louise S. Parent, Pharm.D. "Additional Benefits and Risks of HRT for Osteoporosis." *Drug Topics* 134, no. 3 (February 5, 1990): 68-80.

Sherman, Carl. "Recommends Early Estrogen Therapy for Menopause." *Family Practice News* 23, no. 2 (January 15, 1993).

Stanford, Janet L., Ph.D., et al. "Combined Estrogen and Progestin Hormone Replacement Therapy in Relation to Risk of Breast Cancer in Middle-Aged Women." *Journal of the American Medical Association* 274, no. 2 (July 12, 1995): 137-42.

Steinberg, Karen K., Ph.D., et al. "A Meta-Analysis of the Effect of Estrogen Replacement Therapy on the Risk of Breast Cancer." *Journal of the American Medical Association* 265, no. 15 (April 17, 1991): 1985-90.

Tonouye, Elyse. "Delicate Balance: Estrogen Study Shifts Ground for Women—and for Drug Firms," *Wall Street Journal,* 15 June 1995, sec A, p. 1.

Vassilopoulou-Sellin, Rena, M.D. "Estrogen Replacement Therapy for Breast Cancer Survivors." *Female Patient* 18, no. 8 (August 1993): 41-48.

Wells, Robert G., M.D. "Hormone Replacement Therapy Before Menopause: Is It a Good Idea?" *Postgraduate Medicine* 86, no. 6 (November 1, 1989): 61-71.

INDEX

A

Absolute contraindications, defined, 77, 221

Acne, oral contraceptives and, 39

Acupressure
  defined, 190-191, 221
  hot flashes and, 190-191

Acupuncture
  defined, 190-191, 221
  hot flashes and, 190-191

Adolescence, estrogen and, 18

Adrenal glands, defined, 35-36, 221

Adrenaline, *See* Epinephrine

Age
  breast cancer and, 140, 143-144
  estrogen dose and, 87-88
  menopause and, 17
  perimenopause and, 48-50

Aging, HRT and, 19

Alcohol, osteoporosis and, 106

Alternative therapies
  acupuncture and acupressure, 190-191
  Ayurvedic medicine, 192
  Bach flower remedies, 192
  biofeedback, 191
  Chinese medicine, 192
  homeopathy, 183-184
  naturopathy, 184-187, 189-190
  questions for practitioner, 188-189
  self-help, 192

Alzheimer's disease, estrogen and, 123-124, 209

Amen, *See* Medroxyprogesterone acetate

Amenorrhea, defined, 221

Androgen, defined, 221

Androstenedione, defined, 36, 221

Anemia, iron deficiency, oral contraceptives and, 39

Angina
  defined, 38, 221
  oral contraceptives and, 38

Angiotensin, defined, 82, 222

Anise
  defined, 187, 222
  role, 187

Anti-inflammatory medications, osteoporosis and, 107

Antihypertensives
  defined, 162, 222
  hot flashes and, 162

Appetite, combination HRT and, 76

Artificial menopause, defined, 42, 222

Aspiration endometrial biopsy, defined, 136, 222

Aspirin, thromboembolic disease and, 149

Atherosclerosis, heart disease risk and, 116

Atrophic changes
  defined, 55, 222
  menopause and, 55-56